The book is exceptionally timely and will be of interest to many professionals, students and academics. I am not aware of any other book that covers this important topic. Glenn Laverack brings credibility and kudos having direct experience of health emergencies and seen as a leading academic thinker in health promotion.

— **Dr. James Woodall**
Reader in Health Promotion, Leeds Recltett University

Using specific examples to illustrate broader concepts, this text provides a solid introduction to health promotion in infectious disease outbreaks.

— **Ella Watson-Stryker**
Health Promotion Manager, Médecins Sans Frontières

This book is timely given the current humanitarian and development scenarios in which health promoters and development communicators must work. There is a dire need for reference materials for practitioners which expand upon theoretical/scientific concepts and principles and provide practical, straightforward guidance to professionals working in the field. The increasing amount of public health emergencies, e.g. SARS, Ebola, Zika etc. require professionals to increase their preparedness to respond in outbreak or disaster situations and this book becomes a useful tool for needed action. This is a practical resource for health promotion practitioners involved in responding to disease outbreaks and who are responsible developing behaviour and social change interventions – a definite must read!

— **Dr. Erma Manoncourt**
Vice-President of Membership and Co-Chair Global Working Group on the Social Determinants of Health, IUHPE, Paris, France

Another valuable and informative book by Dr Glenn Laverack, the professor who champions the value of ordinary people and communities, and places them at the centre of best health promotion practice. This is a very welcome text that complements and sometimes challenges the traditional medical, top-down, approaches to disease outbreaks. As the author says, "It is not only about being scientifically right, but also about being real." The book puts communication, education and engagement at its heart, showing how working sensitively with local people, and empowering them to become part of the solution, we can quickly and successfully limit the rapid outbreak of disease and help communities to move forward in a self-directed, sustainable way. Full of contemporary international examples, case studies and helpful short summaries of key points and terminology, this readable text is not only essential for any undergraduate or postgraduate studying health promotion, health protection or public health, it needs to be read by practitioners who are dealing with the immense challenges of international health emergencies now.

— **Dr. Sally Robinson**
Christ Church University

T0199291

# HEALTH PROMOTION IN DISEASE OUTBREAKS AND HEALTH EMERGENCIES

## Glenn Laverack

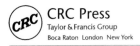

CRC Press
Taylor & Francis Group
Boca Raton London New York

CRC Press is an imprint of the
Taylor & Francis Group, an **informa** business

CRC Press
Taylor & Francis Group
6000 Broken Sound Parkway NW, Suite 300
Boca Raton, FL 33487-2742

© 2018 by Taylor & Francis Group, LLC
CRC Press is an imprint of Taylor & Francis Group, an Informa business

No claim to original U.S. Government works

Printed on acid-free paper

International Standard Book Number-13: 978-1-138-09320-1 (Hardback)
978-1-138-09317-1 (Paperback)

### Library of Congress Cataloging-in-Publication Data

Names: Laverack, Glenn, author.
Title: Health promotion in disease outbreaks and health emergencies / Glenn Laverack.
Description: Boca Raton : CRC Press, [2018] | Includes bibliographical references and index.
Identifiers: LCCN 2017023821 (print) | LCCN 2017024664 (ebook) | ISBN 9781315106885 (Master eBook) | ISBN 9781138093171 (pbk. : alk. paper) | ISBN 9781138093201 (hardback : alk. paper)
Subjects: | MESH: Disease Outbreaks | Health Promotion--organization & administration | Organizations--organization & administration | Community Health Services--organization & administration | Emergencies | Epidemiologic Methods
Classification: LCC RA427.8 (ebook) | LCC RA427.8 (print) | NLM WA 105 | DDC 362.1068--dc23
LC record available at https://lccn.loc.gov/2017023821

**Visit the Taylor & Francis Web site at**
**http://www.taylorandfrancis.com**

**and the CRC Press Web site at**
**http://www.crcpress.com**

# Contents

# List of boxes

## CHAPTER 9

## CHAPTER 10

# List of figures

# Preface

Over the past 20 years, the number of international actors involved in disease outbreak and health emergency responses has dramatically increased. Typically, hundreds of non-government organisations are mobilised alongside the United Nations, government and private sector stakeholders, greatly complicating the coordination of the situation. Concerns about the ease of transmission of communicable diseases across international borders have also dramatically increased, further compounded by the complexity of connections between people that span both geographical and cultural borders.

Health promotion has a key role to play in disease outbreaks and health emergencies by offering bottom-up approaches that actively involve communities by using local expertise and networks in the delivery of the response. A unique aspect of disease outbreaks is that the timeframe of activities is a deciding factor in how many lives are saved and in such circumstances health promotion can be can be quickly integrated as a part of a response. Future global threats to public health may come from one disease such as a new strain of avian influenza or from a combination of person-to-person and vector-borne outbreaks. Whatever the context, health promotion will play a crucial role in rapid data collection, communication, community engagement, rumour management and conflict resolution. It will also play a strong role in the promotion of vaccination, in changing behaviours and in helping to build a dialogue to address the constraints that create an unsafe environment. In the post-outbreak period, health promotion will help survivors by increasing awareness about available facilities and by promoting the use of counselling and welfare initiatives. Health promotion will help to build social support networks and to counter stigma and isolation and to assist with rehabilitation services for people with disabilities.

Community engagement is an especially important activity to help others to address the risks that are caused by an outbreak. Communication is a crucial step in this approach to promote positive health behaviours such as hygiene promotion that prevents disease transmission. The guiding principle is to help people to make informed choices and to give them more control to take their own actions such as community-built latrines. The critical point is that disease outbreaks can only be addressed by helping people to empower themselves rather than by simply trying to change their behaviour. The advantage of empowerment is that it can strengthen the individual, the family and the community. Empowerment increases autonomy and personal skills and gives people the control they need to achieve healthier, safer lives.

Top-down tactics have had a questionable effect, potentially worsening a disease outbreak, and contributing to a greater social and economic burden. A key concern is whether the lessons offered in previous disease outbreaks have been truly learned, or whether a top-down agenda will continue to dominate the disease outbreak responses of the future. Health promotion can make an important contribution because it recognises the value of a bottom-up approach that can help response agencies to understand a more appropriate way forward. Involving everyone, most importantly those people directly affected, is crucial to the success of any response when the next outbreak or emergency inevitably occurs.

## THE PURPOSE OF THIS BOOK

The purpose of this book is to provide a practical guide to the valuable role that health promotion can play in disease outbreaks and health emergencies. This is an exciting and emerging sub-professional field within health promotion that requires a balanced set of competencies combining the latest evidence with the best practices. The book has been written in an easy-to-read style that has a crossover appeal to the students, teachers and practitioners of health promotion, public health and other allied professions. I have used a good deal of my own personal international experience as well as consulting with many others about the most relevant content for the book. Through this book, I want to inspire the reader to think beyond the traditional role of health promotion and to understand how he or she can have a meaningful role in disease outbreaks and health emergencies.

## THE ORGANIZATION OF THIS BOOK

This book is divided into three parts that comprehensively cover the role that health promoters have in disease outbreaks and health emergencies. The first part of the book, Chapters 1–5, provides a detailed overview of the role of health promotion beginning in Chapter 1 by setting the context of this new and exciting professional field. The differentiation between top-down and bottom-up approaches and an identification of the key stakeholders are discussed. Chapters 2–5 then cover key areas of health promotion practice. Chapter 2 discusses quantitative and qualitative methods to collect information quickly and effectively using rapid assessment techniques, working in a cross-cultural context and the relevance of anthropology. Chapter 3 covers communication for both behaviour change and empowerment and a variety of reliable communication approaches that can be applied in disease outbreaks. Chapter 4 discusses the distinct role of risk communication, fear-based interventions and the importance of working with volunteers and lay health workers in disease outbreaks. Chapter 5 provides a framework for community engagement as a practical seven-step approach and a discussion of the role of community engagement in clinical trials. Community empowerment and health activism are also discussed, as these processes are often a result of community engagement and can lead to greater collective action. The second part of this book, Chapters 6–8, directly addresses the role of health promotion in different types of disease outbreaks that are transmitted either person to person or are vector borne. Chapter 6 is devoted to the Ebola virus disease, the first disease to be declared a global security threat by the United Nations, and a health emergency that can offer valuable lessons for other events in the future. Chapter 7 covers person-to-person disease transmission with a particular focus on avian influenza, cholera, polio and the Middle East respiratory syndrome outbreaks. Chapter 8 covers vector-borne transmission with a particular focus on the Zika virus, Nipah disease, chikungunya disease and yellow fever. Some diseases can be controlled through vaccines, and Chapter 8 discusses the role of health promotion in vaccination programmes. The third part of this book covers the role of health promotion in specialist areas of work in disease outbreaks and health emergencies. Chapter 9 covers the management of community rumours, community resistance, violence and protests, the management of quarantines and coordinating security issues with military personnel. Chapter 10 discusses the role of health promotion in the post-outbreak response including working with survivors to address stigma and isolation, building networks, counselling and helping people to cope with disabilities. A full reference list, index and glossary of terms are provided at the end of the book.

# Acknowledgements

---

I would like to acknowledge the many people with whom I have exchanged ideas and experiences. In particular, I would like to thank Gaya Gamhewage for her initial encouragement, Krystle Lai and Ella Watson-Stryker for their review of the draft manuscript and Erma Manoncourt for being my inspiration.

To my family, Elizabeth, Ben, Holly and Rebecca just because I love them.

# Health promotion, disease outbreaks and health emergencies

Over the past 20 years the number of international agencies involved in disease outbreak and health emergency responses has increased significantly. In the aftermath of the 2010 earthquake in Haiti, for example, several hundred international non-government organisations were mobilised alongside the United Nations, government, and the private sectors, greatly increasing the complexity of the situation. The growing number of such events has placed pressure on the availability of funding opportunities. At the same time, there has been a realisation that the goal of involving communities has not succeeded, yet such involvement is crucial to the success of a response (Tellier and Roche 2016). The ease of the transmission of diseases between countries is a major issue, and the response in one country cannot be separated from that of another country because connections between people and organisations span geographic and cultural borders (Naidoo and Wills 2009). The outbreak of the Ebola virus disease, for example, was exasperated by the cross-border movement of people as well as by already fragile healthcare systems.

> The goal of health promotion in disease outbreaks and health emergencies is to involve and enable people to gain more control to have healthier and safer lives.

## HEALTH PROMOTION

Health promotion is a set of principles involving equity and participation and a practice that encompasses communication, capacity building and politically orientated activities. The definition provided in the Ottawa Charter for Health Promotion is still the most universally recognised as 'a process of enabling people to increase control over, and to improve, their health' (World Health Organization 1986). Health promotion represents a social and political process that not only embraces actions directed at strengthening the skills and knowledge of individuals, but also action directed towards changing sociocultural, environmental and economic conditions that have an impact on health.

A unique aspect of disease outbreaks and health emergencies is that the situation can change quickly and also the speed at which activities are delivered can be a deciding factor in preventing the transmission of an infection. In a disease outbreak, health promoters are practitioners who incorporate some aspect of communication and community engagement in their everyday work. These workers include medical personnel, health educators, community mobilisers, social workers, trainers and managers. Health promoters play a key role to quickly deliver approaches that government and non-government agencies alike can utilise as a part of any response. Health promotion is also a core responsibility for government services in many countries and can be quickly integrated in a disease outbreak response by providing local expertise and a basic infrastructure for the delivery of a range of communications and other activities. The role of the health promoter also includes data collection, communication, community capacity building and engagement, rumour and resistance management, stigma recognition, survivor support and provision of social support to families and communities.

Behaviour change communication, Communication for Development (C4D) and hygiene promotion interventions help to prevent person-to-person disease transmission by targeting specific knowledge and skills, such as hand-washing with soap. In controlling vector-borne diseases, health promotion uses health education messaging so that people know how best to protect themselves and their communities. The purpose is to motivate people to change high-risk behaviours by giving them improved skills and self-confidence. The focus on individual responsibility must avoid 'victim-blaming', that is, making people feel guilty about their state of health even though certain risk factors are outside of their control, such as not having access to a bed net to protect themselves against mosquitoes. The role of health education departments at the national level is to design learning materials and provide training, instruction and skills development. The guiding principle is to help people to make informed choices to modify their behaviours and to avoid risks.

> Health promotion can provide a range of educational and skills development activities that are essential to help people to empower themselves during a disease outbreak.

# DISEASE OUTBREAKS AND HEALTH EMERGENCIES

Endemic refers to the usual prevalence of a disease in a population within a geographic area. An outbreak refers to an increase, often sudden, in the number of cases of a disease above the endemic level in the population. An outbreak can occur within a restricted geographic area or it may extend over a much broader

## BOX 1.1: The International Health Regulations

The International Health Regulations (IHR) were enforced on 15 June 2007 with the purpose and scope to 'prevent, protect against, control and provide a public health response to the international spread of disease in ways that are commensurate with and restricted to public health risks, and which avoid unnecessary interference with international traffic and trade' (World Health Organization 2016f, article 2). The IHR help the international community prevent and respond to acute public health risks that have the potential to cross borders and threaten people worldwide. The IHR are an international legal instrument that is binding on 196 countries that have agreed to build their capacities to detect, assess and report public health events. The IHR are not limited to specific diseases and also apply to new and emerging public health risks to have long-lasting relevance to international responses. However, there are four communicable diseases that require notification in all circumstances: (1) any laboratory-confirmed case of a recent human infection caused by an influenza A virus with the potential to cause a pandemic; (2) a case of poliomyelitis due to wild-type poliovirus in a stool specimen collected from the suspected case or from a close contact of the suspected case; (3) a case of severe acute respiratory syndrome (SARS) from an individual with laboratory confirmation of infection with the coronavirus (CoV) who either fulfils the clinical case definition of SARS or has worked in a laboratory working with live SARS-CoV or storing clinical specimens infected with SARS-CoV; (4) any confirmed case of smallpox (World Health Organization 2016c).

area for a prolonged period. A single case of a disease not normally present in the population can also constitute an outbreak, for example, as for the poliovirus, and must be reported and investigated. A disease outbreak may result from a recent increase in the amount or virulence of the disease, a recent introduction of the disease into a setting where it has not been before, an enhanced mode of transmission so that more susceptible persons are exposed, a change in the susceptibility of the host response to the disease, and/or factors that increase host exposure or involve a new means of entry into the population (Kelsey et al. 1986).

A pandemic is an outbreak that occurs on a scale crossing international boundaries, usually affecting a large number of people (Porta 2014). The severe acute respiratory syndrome (SARS) virus, for example, killed 800 people in the Asia-Pacific region in 2002 and was contained by using rigorous sanitation procedures and barrier nursing techniques such as latex gloves, face masks and disposable gowns when in contact with infected patients (Doherty 2013). An emergency is a state that demands a response as an extraordinary measure. A 'state of emergency' is declared and lifted by those in authority and is dependent on the scale, timing, unpredictability and capabilities of existing services to respond. All emergencies have a health aspect that can be caused by natural disasters, civil emergencies, disease outbreaks and the release of hazardous materials into the environment. A health emergency specially occurs when the consequences have the potential to overwhelm the capabilities of the health system to contain the problem (Nelson et al. 2007). Disease outbreaks and health emergencies are closely connected, and this book uses the term 'disease outbreaks' to cover both contexts.

## Disease prevention

Disease prevention deals with individuals and populations exhibiting identifiable risk factors, often associated with different risk behaviours (World Health Organization 1998) to prevent the occurrence of a disease and to reduce its consequences once established. Health promotion is concerned with the primary, secondary and tertiary stages of disease prevention. Primary prevention is directed towards preventing the initial onset of ill health by, for example, the detection of risk factors and appropriate health messages. Secondary prevention seeks to change unhealthy behaviour or to shorten the period of ill health and its progression (e.g. educational and motivational strategies to increase the use of hand-washing). Tertiary prevention seeks to limit the effects of a condition and enhance a person's quality of life (e.g. effective rehabilitation therapy) (Naidoo and Wills 2009).

Communicable disease, also called infectious and transmissible disease, comprises clinically evident illnesses resulting from pathogenic agents in an individual or population group and can include viruses, bacteria, fungi and protozoa. A communicable disease is transmitted from a source, such as from one person to another or from a vector to a person. Identifying the means of transmission is important in helping people to understand how to prevent the disease outbreak and focuses on controlling or eliminating the cause of transmission, the vector or high-risk behaviours. Sometimes, this identification can be done using a physical method (e.g. a bed net to prevent being bitten by a mosquito) or a vaccine to reduce the effect of the disease (e.g. for cholera). Surveillance is particularly important because of the infectious nature and the rapid spread of communicable diseases. Information that is used for surveillance comes from various sources, including reported cases of communicable diseases, hospital admissions, laboratory reports, population surveys, reports of absence from school or work, and reported causes of death (Public Health Agency of Canada 2013).

Screening is designed to identify disease, thus enabling prevention, management and treatment to reduce mortality. Mass screening covers a whole population or a subgroup, irrespective of the risk status of the individual. High-risk or selective screening is conducted among individuals of a risk population. The selection of screening tests for an individual depends on age, sex, family history and risk factors for certain diseases. Screening can show positive for those without a disease, called a false positive, or negative for people who have the condition, called a false negative. Over-diagnosis can also make screening seem successful by finding abnormalities, even though they are sometimes harmless, and are counted as 'lives saved' rather than as healthy people with a manageable condition (Raffle and Muir Gray 2007). Health promotion plays an important preventive role in the screening process including education and counselling interventions and behaviour change to combat, for example, the spread of sexually transmitted diseases through condom use or ensuring a drug regime is completed such as to combat the transmission of tuberculosis.

Drug resistance is the reduction in the effectiveness of a treatment because of the resistance by some pathogens. The development of antibiotic resistance, for example, derives from some drugs targeting only specific bacterial proteins, and therefore any mutation in these proteins interferes with its destructive effect.

## BOX 1.2: Drug resistance and tuberculosis

XDR-TB is an abbreviation for extensively drug-resistant (XDR) tuberculosis (TB) that is resistant to at least four of the core anti-TB drugs. Multidrug-resistant (MDR-TB) and XDR-TB both take substantially longer to treat than ordinary drug-susceptible TB and require the use of second-line anti-TB drugs, which are more expensive and have more side effects. Three countries carry the major burden of MDR-TB—India, China and the Russian Federation— together accounting for nearly half of all cases globally. The risk of spread of MDR-TB and XDR-TB increases where there is a high concentration of TB bacteria, such as can occur in overcrowded living conditions, hospitals or prisons. Health promoters have an important role to work with individuals, families and communities to provide information, counselling and material support to enable patients to continue taking all their drug treatment as prescribed. No doses should be missed and, above all, treatment should be taken right through to completion (National Research Council 2003).

It has been the lack of a committed strategy by governments and the pharmaceutical industries that has allowed organisms to develop resistance at a rate that has been faster than new drug development can occur. Drug resistance can sometimes be minimised by using a combination of multiple drugs, for example, in the treatment of tuberculosis (National Research Council 2003).

## Super-spreaders and disease outbreaks

A 'super-spreader' is a host, such as a human, that is infected with a disease and that in turn infects disproportionally more secondary contacts than other hosts also infected with the same disease. Super-spreaders may or may not be asymptomatic. It is often assumed that infected individuals within a population have equal chances of transmitting an infection to others. The 20/80 rule in a disease outbreak applies when approximately 20% of infected individuals are responsible for 80% of transmission. Super-spreading occurs when fewer individuals account for a much higher percentage of the transmission and the majority of other individuals infect relatively few secondary contacts. For example, it has been estimated that in Freetown, Sierra Leone, as many as 61% of cases were caused by only 3% of infected people (Gallagher 2017).

It is uncertain what actually makes some people disproportionately more likely to transmit a disease than others. Super-spreading events are shaped by multiple factors including co-infection with another pathogen, immune suppression, changes in airflow dynamics, delayed and inter-hospital admission, misdiagnosis and differences in the host–pathogen relationship (Rothman et al. 2008). Predicting and identifying super-spreaders can have significant health

---

**BOX 1.3: Super-spreading and the SARS outbreak**

The first outbreak of severe acute respiratory syndrome (SARS) occurred in 2002 in Guangdong Province in southeastern China, followed by an outbreak in Hong Kong. A doctor in Guangdong who had treated SARS cases contracted the virus and was symptomatic but travelled to Hong Kong to attend a family wedding. He infected 16 other hotel guests who then travelled to Canada, Singapore, Taiwan and Vietnam, spreading SARS and starting the risk of a global outbreak. Another case during the same outbreak involved a man who was admitted to a hospital with suspected coronary heart disease, chronic renal failure and type II diabetes. He had been in contact with a patient known to have SARS, and shortly after his admission he developed a fever, a cough and a sore throat. He was transferred to another hospital for treatment, but his SARS symptoms became worse. This one person transmitted the disease to 33 other patients in 2 days and eventually died. The SARS outbreak caused 8273 cases and 775 deaths and was spread to 37 countries (Shen et al. 2004).

promotion implications for targeting messaging and the mobilisation of community self-management of cases.

The 2015 Middle East respiratory syndrome (MERS) coronavirus (MERS-CoV) outbreak in South Korea is an example of when a single imported case, a 68-year-old male, with a recent travel history to several Middle Eastern countries, started a disease outbreak. A complex combination of factors played a role in the transmission of the disease from the single super-spreader including environmental factors such as the close proximity of other susceptible hosts and the airflow dynamics within an enclosed area. Hospitals, enclosed housing complexes and mass transportation, such as airplanes, facilitate super-spreader events as well as 'doctor shopping', that is, going to multiple hospitals to treat the same ailments which was observed with the MERS-CoV outbreak (Wong et al. 2015). In the West African Ebola outbreak, most cases had a relatively short infectious period and generated low numbers of secondary infections; however, a small number had longer infectious periods and generated more infections. This was especially pronounced in children under 15 years old and adults over 45 years old. The reasons for this super-spreading were unclear but may be attributed to behavioural factors, sometimes not even the infected cases but rather to the people around them. This may have been related to the nature of the transmission of the Ebola virus disease combined with specific cultural practices regarding the care for the young and elderly members of the family (Gallagher 2017).

Anthropological information is key to interpret complex cultural situations and how they might apply to super-spreader events in a disease outbreak. The role of health promotion is to communicate how these complex cultural situations can affect people's health and the health of others and to provide information and skills during an outbreak to help change high-risk behaviours. This is best achieved by developing a dialogue to identify, at both an individual and a community level, when high-risk situations occur and the collaborative actions that are required to resolve them.

## PROGRAMME MANAGEMENT

Health promotion can be delivered as a programme, a project, an intervention or a set of specific activities. I have used the term 'programme' in this book to cover the range of different types and stages of the delivery. Programme management requires a workforce with multi-disciplinary skills including administrators; human resource personnel; and budgeting, training, procurement and reporting experts. The purpose is to ensure that the programme is delivered on time, on budget and in accordance with its aims and objectives. Consequently, there has been a reluctance to transfer responsibility to other partners who are perceived as having a different set of skills (e.g. community members), even though they are expected to cooperate with and contribute towards the programme. Managers can underestimate the assets of local partners, and this can be further confounded when the programme involves cross-cultural aspects and does not consider the resilience of cultural values and the distrust felt by people who are excluded by the programme (Leach 1994).

> At the heart of a successful outbreak response is who controls the way in which the disease control programme is designed and implemented.

## Top-down and bottom-up styles of management

Top-down and bottom-up styles of management are ideal types of practice that demonstrate important differences in relation to the delivery of health promotion programmes. Top-down management occurs when the programme needs are defined by the outside agent, the top structures of the system, and are delivered down to the recipients. The agency also exercises control of financial and other material resources over the programme. Top-down is a form of dominance in which control is exerted through the design, implementation and evaluation of the programme. The agency pushes down a predefined agenda, often with the best intention to improve health, and this can be problematic when it creates a 'bottom-up versus top-down tension' as communities struggle to also get their needs addressed. The approach can be used as an instrument of control through performance measurement, the achievement of targets and by providing feedback about the operational elements of the implementation. Top-down approaches commonly use standard protocols and operating procedures that do not include input from communities. Top-down responses typically make the incorrect assumption that the agency possesses the knowledge needed to halt an outbreak and that the local population does not have to be involved other than to cooperate in the delivery of the response. For example, in cross-border areas of high mobility where movement patterns were based on ancient trade routes and used for family visits across porous international borders (McConnell 2014), some agencies have tried unsuccessfully to police people rather than to collaborate with local leaders.

Bottom-up management is the reverse in which the local population identifies its own needs and communicates these to the top structures. Community engagement is closely linked to a health promotion practice that recognises the value of including local people in planning and implementation and that seeks to listen to and respond to the expressed needs of communities. The role of the management is to systematically build the capacity, knowledge and skills of the local partners to be able to be involved in the programme. One of the first steps towards achieving this goal is to have clearly defined roles and responsibilities of everyone involved in the programme. For example, during the planning stage the needs of local partners should be assessed and included in the aims of the programme. A bottom-up style of management places the focus on capacity building and participatory methods and moves practice away from conventional 'expert'-driven approaches. This means a fundamental shift between the agency and the beneficiaries of the programme, a shift where control over decisions is more equitably distributed.

In a disease outbreak or health emergency, the health promoter should not have to make a choice between a top-down and a bottom-up management approach. Both are necessary in a response. Top-down approaches are able to implement activities quickly to slow down the chain of transmission. Bottom-up approaches are essential to ensure community involvement in the delivery of the response. However, the top-down approach can become dominant because some agencies are unwilling to relinquish control; as a consequence, this can lead to community resistance, rumours and poor cooperation.

## PROGRAMME DESIGN CONSIDERATIONS

Disease outbreaks require planning across all sectors, including agriculture, education, housing, transport and health. At a national level, this would involve a whole of government approach that focuses on public communication, coordination and the efficient delivery of resources. Disease outbreak responses can be most effective when they allow the involvement of all the different stakeholders and the various financial, material and human resources that they are able to make available.

## Coordination

Establishing and maintaining coordination mechanisms for an outbreak response is an important priority to ensure appropriate representation and input from all stakeholders representing agency, government and civil society groups. Political leadership at national and local levels is crucial, and the responsibility of coordinating the response should not be left to the local health authorities nor should it be dominated by a top-down approach. The United Nations, for example, did learn from its earlier mistakes during the Ebola response to better engage with communities. There was no excuse not to actively involve local people; however, bottom-up approaches were not widely implemented at the beginning of the response (Laverack and Manoncourt 2015).

The United Nations Mission for Ebola Emergency Response (UNMEER) was the first UN emergency health mission, established on 19 September 2014 and closed on 31 July 2015. To establish unity of purpose among the many stakeholders in support of the nationally led efforts in the three affected countries, the UNMEER had a major role in coordinating the key programme activities:

- Case finding and contact tracing: Sufficient teams were recruited, trained and logistically supported in every district to ensure that all cases are found rapidly and that all affected communities or contacts were identified and monitored daily.
- Case management: Sufficient treatment, transit/referral and care centres were built and staffed with trained personnel to ensure all suspect, probable and confirmed cases can be safely isolated and cared for on the same day that they are identified.
- Community engagement and social mobilisation: Efforts were made to ensure that all religious, traditional and community leaders were engaged at the national and local levels, supported by a social mobilisation network to deliver messages to each household.
- Safe and dignified burials: Sufficient district and sub-district level burial teams were identified, trained and equipped to provide safe and dignified, same-day burials and remuneration for work.

The key health promotion activities of community engagement and social mobilisation were led by the United Nations Children's Fund (UNICEF) as a technical 'pillar' in the three affected countries. The pillar was led by the ministries of health and the corresponding health promotion units with support from United Nations agencies and civil society organisations. The main function of the community engagement and social mobilisation pillar was to coordinate efforts for behaviour change as well as to measure and report on key performance indicators. C4D was a key strategy (see Chapter 3) to influence and implement policies; to mobilise civil society; to actively help to empower households and communities; and to identify problems, propose solutions, and then act upon them (Gillespie et al. 2016).

## Time frame

A unique aspect of disease outbreaks and health emergencies is that the time frame of activities is a deciding factor in how many lives are saved through preventing the transmission of the infection. For health promotion, the initial period is when the community and outbreak response is at its most vulnerable, and working quickly and efficiently is very important. The local community serves as the first responders, and therefore the programme must be operational quickly to build trust and to obtain community permission for medical and disease control activities. Later, systems and procedures need to be in place to limit the spread of the disease through effective communication about the risks, for example, by using local radio and community educators. A more coordinated approach is established, and agencies can focus on the quality of the response and can shift to increasing training and engagement with a broader range of stakeholders to be involved in surveillance, contact tracing and the promotion of community-led activities such as improved sanitation.

> In a disease outbreak the situation can change rapidly and budget flexibility is essential.

## Programme budget

The programme budget is usually itemised using 'budget headings' in regard to specific costs such as administration, training, technical services, materials, equipment and transport. The planned resources are provided over specific periods such as monthly, quarterly, six monthly or annually to cover the total programme duration. Traditionally, there is little flexibility in the programme budget, and once it has been approved it is unlikely to be modified to meet changing expectations. In a disease outbreak the situation can change rapidly and budget flexibility is essential. A percentage of funds can be used to allow unexpected and informal activities to be implemented. Alternatively, the programme management can use a percentage of the budget as a contingency for unforeseeable circumstances that arise as the programme develops.

## Monitoring and evaluation

Monitoring is a periodically recurring task beginning in the planning stage of a programme and allows results, processes and experiences to be documented. The information acquired through monitoring helps to better understand the ways in which the programme has developed over time and how this development can be improved in the future. Process evaluation aims to understand how the programme has been delivered, what actually happened and how people reacted to it. A process evaluation describes the strengths and weaknesses of a programme and engages with the key partners to identify why it has or has not worked in practice (Nutbeam and Bauman 2011).

> Process evaluation is sometimes not well performed or is even omitted because agencies are expected to deliver activities quickly during a disease outbreak.

Outcome evaluation aims to assess whether the programme has achieved its goals and any longer term impact and is usually set against predetermined targets or outcomes. Health targets require an estimate of current and future trends in relation to change in the distribution of an indicator and an understanding of the potential to change the distribution of the indicator in the population. Health outcomes are usually assessed using indicators that can be used to describe one or more measurable aspects of the health of an individual or population over the programme period. Health indicators include the measurement of illness or disease, or positive aspects of health such as behaviours which are related to reducing risk. Process and outcome indicators should be used together to provide a holistic evaluation of the health promotion programme (World Health Organization 1998).

# HUMAN RESOURCES FOR HEALTH IN DISEASE OUTBREAKS

Human resources for health can be defined as all people engaged in actions whose primary intent is to enhance health. Human resources for health deals with the planning, development, performance, management, staff retention, research and development for the healthcare sector (World Health Organization 2006b). Health workers involved in disease outbreaks include doctors, nurses, midwives, allied health professionals, social workers, health communicators, support staff and health supply chain managers. There is a shortage of health workers such as doctors and nurses worldwide, but this shortage is most severe in regions where disease outbreaks often occur such as in West Africa (World Health Organization 2006a). There is also a mal-distribution of skilled health workers which can lead to localised shortages in remote and rural areas within countries. Policies for the recruitment and retention in rural and remote areas need to combine different packages of interventions according to the factors influencing the health workers' decision and match their preferences and expectations influencing their employment decisions (Araujo and Maeda 2013). The future challenges for human resources in outbreak responses include staff mobilisation to address emerging health issues, new skills and relevant competencies. Special skills required by health promoters include coordinated planning, risk communication, rapid community mobilisation and self-management approaches. The tasks required must be integrated into national response systems and ongoing health training.

## Staff deployment in disease outbreaks

The deployment of health promotion personnel into disease outbreak responses usually follows a systematic process of pre-deployment, deployment and post-deployment activities.

Pre-deployment: The health promoter receives a pre-deployment package containing key technical documents, takes part in briefings and teleconferences with in-country focal points and receives a terms of reference to outline the main tasks and deliverables. Pre-service education, training and mentorship are important short-term strategies to strengthen human resources and institutional capacity. Health promotion staff retention and performance at local and national levels can also be enhanced by improving their remuneration and working conditions, addressing the reasons for low deployment, investing in infrastructure improvement, ensuring the provision of equipment and supplies and improving supervision.

Standard tasks in the terms of reference for the health promoter in an outbreak response include the following:

- Coordinate with the government/Ministry of Health plans and strategies
- Use outbreak response standard operating procedures
- Assess communication needs and existing capacity at the country level
- Report to relevant agencies involved in health promotion in the outbreak response
- Collate or conduct knowledge, attitude and practice survey data for the target audience
- Provide technical support to other outbreak response teams

The deliverables include the following:

- Prepare a communication and community engagement strategy for the outbreak response
- Provide timely monitoring calls and reports
- Provide a final report and recommendations including a briefing with colleagues and relevant technical staff

Deployment: The health promoter will take part in regular stakeholder meetings and in briefing calls with the employing agency at the headquarters and/or the regional, district and community levels. The health promoter will also be expected to provide periodic monitoring reports and to deliver the tasks in the terms of reference in order to achieve the required deliverables.

Post-deployment: Concluding the deployment, the health promoter will usually be expected to provide a final report and a post-deployment satisfaction survey or debriefing.

## Professional competencies for health promotion

Professional competencies for health promotion in disease outbreaks include a combination of knowledge, skills and values that enable an individual to perform a set of tasks to an appropriate standard. Core competencies also provide a set of standards by which the workforce can determine what a 'professional' practice is and can be used to set parameters for staff development, recruitment and performance standards. Core competencies include communication strategies; however, for some health workers this is only a small part of their daily work, such as for a nurse who undertakes a mix of clinical practice and health education. It is the responsibility of health promoters to select which specialist competencies they feel are most relevant to their work in an outbreak context (Laverack 2007). Key competencies are given below, and although not exhaustive they provide a guide of what is required to deliver in the disease outbreak response.

---

**BOX 1.4: Key competencies for health promotion in disease outbreaks**

1. Programme design, management, implementation and evaluation: The ability to plan effective health promotion programmes, including the management of resources and personnel involving an understanding of programme cycles, budgeting and the planning and evaluation of bottom-up approaches.
2. Coordination and delivery of effective communication strategies: Communication strategies are an integral part of disease outbreak responses to increase knowledge levels and to raise awareness and involve the coordination of different stakeholders, the identification of the targeted individuals, groups and communities, and the use of communication techniques such as one-to-one communication, print materials and social media.
3. Facilitating skills: Training, for example, for skills development, usually within a workshop setting, is a key part of many programmes. Good facilitation skills are essential for health promoters and are an important part of programme delivery.
4. Community engagement and capacity-building skills: Community engagement and capacity building are central to a range of strategies to help people self-manage their own circumstances at individual,

family and community levels and to gain more control of the situation affecting their health and lives.

5. Translating findings into practical recommendations: The translation of research and other data collection findings into practical recommendations is often a missing link and can be overcome by improved competencies to interpret information and to communicate this to the appropriate programme manager.

## KEY STAKEHOLDERS IN DISEASE OUTBREAKS AND HEALTH EMERGENCIES

Stakeholder identification is important because it has real benefits for the level of participation and for sustainable outcomes. Programmes that do not involve key stakeholders run the real risk of not achieving their goals. The involvement of stakeholders in the planning process is also critical to promote multi-sectoral action for disease prevention and control. Stakeholders are people and organisations that have some interest or influence in the disease outbreak and can therefore change as the situation develops over time. Stakeholders include the population that will be approached to participate, as well as others who are not physically located where the response takes place (UNAIDS 2007). The process of stakeholder identification begins with an analysis of the main individuals and organisations, within health and other sectors, whose work is related to the disease outbreak. The key stakeholders can be broadly categorised into the following sectors: community; non-government sector, including the private sector; faith-based organisations (FBOs); government services; and United Nations agencies.

## Community

It is important to think beyond the customary view of a community as a place where people live, for example, a neighbourhood, because these people are often just an aggregate of non-connected people. Communities have both a social and a geographic characteristic and consist of individuals with dynamic relations that organise into groups to take action towards achieving shared goals. Within the geographic dimensions of 'community', individuals may belong to several different 'interest' groups at the same time. Interest groups exist as a legitimate means by which individuals can find a 'voice' and are able to participate to pursue their interests in the disease outbreak (Zakus and Lysack 1998). Interest groups can be organised around a variety of social activities or can address a local concern, for example, poor access to ambulance services. This group includes both members of the public within the area of the outbreak with whom engagement is essential and members of the public outside the area of the outbreak to prevent the spread of the disease.

## Non-government sector

'Non-government organisation' is a term used to cover all not-for-profit organisations, voluntary, community, charities and social non-government associations. Non-government organisations want to offer support during a disease outbreak and have an extensive network at the local level that can facilitate message and resource distribution. Building alliances with these partners early on and assigning clearly defined responsibilities can significantly contribute to an organised and efficient response. Business, trade and industry will want to avoid the loss of revenue and liability during an outbreak or health emergency and will want to take steps to protect the health of their employees. Private sector organisations and businesses can provide resources, equipment or relevant expertise, for example, corporate donations of personal protective equipment, cleaning supplies or medical supplies for an outbreak.

## Faith-based organisations

Faith plays an important role in people's lives. People listen to their faith leaders and often come to places of worship for a source of reliable information, compassion and social support. Faith leaders also play an important role in communities where they have significant trust and respect. Communities are often more trusting of informal networks that include religious leaders and faith-based community health, social, and pastoral services. Once they became involved, faith leaders can also play a transformational role by working with communities, for example, by accompanying families to funerals and by conducting modified religious practices, to encourage people to comply with the need for safe and dignified burials (CAFOD 2015). FBOs often have a role as a secondary stakeholder not only in disseminating information but also in helping to convince communities to undertake preventive measures.

During the initial phase of an outbreak response, there can be a poor understanding by government and international agencies about the diversity of religious communities and the role of FBOs. This can delay the establishment of collaborative partnerships and the mobilisation of assets such as knowledge, trust, infrastructure and social networks. Christian Health Associations, for example, were already active in Liberia and Sierra Leone in the early stages of the Ebola outbreak and engaged with volunteers, provided medical supplies and organised the training of pastors, the texting of health messages to congregations and the care for orphans (Marshall and Smith 2015). FBOs formed the 'Social Mobilization and Respectful Burials Through Faith-Based Alliance Consortium', which played pivotal role in supervising burial teams. FBOs also supported negotiations for the access and protection of health workers from government and non-government organisations that were previously attacked by community members due to feelings of fear and resistance (Greyling et al. 2016).

FBOs have argued that the messages they use replace fear with feelings of hope and are delivered with compassion in a way that provides encouragement. They claim that the holistic way in which faith leaders are able to engage with people

> **BOX 1.5: World Council of Churches**
>
> The World Council of Churches has a network of 345 member churches, representing more than 560 million Christians in 110 countries. The faith-based communities play an important role in mobilising the population, providing information, addressing stigma, and providing compassionate burial ceremonies and psychosocial and pastoral counselling to survivors, family members and healthcare workers. The World Council of Churches is well established and often has the trust of the communities in which it works and can be an important partner agency in outbreak responses (World Council of Churches 2015).

from both a technical and religious perspective enables deep-seated traditional behaviour changes to occur. The role of health promotion is to assist FBOs to ensure that the messages they use are consistent and correct. This assistance is needed because there have been concerns about the self-serving motivations of some FBOs that has sometimes made government and United Nations agencies hesitant to partner with them; however, their long-term presence and community-based networks are increasingly being recognised as important to a holistic response to a disease outbreak or health emergency (Greyling et al. 2016).

> Community- and faith-based organisations are an essential partner to a holistic and effective disease outbreak response.

## Government services

The local, regional or national government authorities are the starting point for planning and establishing health services, for example, the Ministry of Health, hospitals, clinics, public health and health promotion services. The Ministry of Foreign Affairs is important because diseases can transcend national boundaries and ensuring cooperation, information exchange and planning between countries will increase the likelihood of success. The starting point of the outbreak response is at the national level to provide the information needs of all stakeholders: (a) those affected by or at risk of the outbreak and (b) those responding to the outbreak as they carry out their work.

To bring the different stakeholders together in a common platform, at the national level, different clusters or pillars can be established by the national government in collaboration with supporting agencies. The pillars meet on a regular basis to plan, coordinate and mediate between agencies and to facilitate the delivery of activities in a rapidly changing situation. Healthcare professionals involved in the response are concerned with ensuring that treatment and prevention protocols are followed and that resources are provided. The health promotion or health education unit, often within the Ministry of Health, plays a key role in planning and coordinating communication activities, community mobilisation and improving participation in the outbreak response such as promoting the use of vaccination services.

## United Nations agencies

The task of managing an outbreak is initially left to national governments and non-government organisations; but as the emergency continues to accelerate, and the disease poses a greater threat, an international or global response led by the United Nations may be triggered. The situation can be complex, requiring extraordinary measures to control and contain the transmission of a disease through collaboration and coordination between the international community, government and local populations. With so many organisations being deployed on the ground, the first priority is sufficient healthcare facilities such as hospital beds for patients. Once this is met, the focus shifts to other services such as surveillance, case management, safe burials, contact tracing and crucially to community engagement and social mobilisation.

United Nations agencies such as UNICEF can provide an operational cadre of 'social mobilisers' that are usually community health workers that exist in the country, for example, from government or other initiatives, and that can be employed in a disease outbreak as fieldworkers at the district and local levels. Their purpose is to assist with communication, training, stakeholder engagement, and the mobilisation and coordination of targeted interventions such as community quarantines and behaviour change communication.

# 2

# Collecting information effectively and quickly

---

## KEY POINTS

- Quickly translating on-the-ground information into practice is not always possible because it requires a specific skill set that can be lacking in a disease outbreak response.
- Communities are open to rational discussion and health promoters are well placed to engage with them to offer advice that is based on sound evidence.
- It is essential to have a coordination mechanism to track and to share the findings of all data collection and research that is carried out in the response.
- Good facilitation is crucial to collecting information but can be hard to find and must be constantly monitored for quality of delivery.
- Participatory data collection that does not offer people the means to transform information into action is not empowering.

## AN EVIDENCE-BASED PRACTICE FOR HEALTH PROMOTION

Health promotion practice involves the use of the best available scientific evidence and the knowledge and experiences of the practitioner, professional partners and the community. An evidence-based practice should go beyond research and use the skills and experience of the professional alongside values that inform decision-making and programme design in the local population (Hoffman et al. 2013). It is not only about being scientifically right but also about being real in practice.

The movement to develop an evidence-based practice has consistently used a scientific discourse in which the information derived from randomised controlled trials (RCTs) has been the most highly rated. The evidence is rated as follows: (1) meta-analysis of RCTs; (2) at least one RCT; (3) one randomised study without randomisation; (4) one other types of quasi-experimental study; (5) non-experimental descriptive studies (comparative, case–control); and (6) expert committees or the opinions or clinical experience of respected authorities (Marks 2002). The choice of evidence has favoured the quasi-experiment of the RCT, although this is not considered to be the most appropriate for professional fields such as health promotion.

> Quickly translating on-the-ground data into practice is not always possible because it requires a skill set that can be lacking in an outbreak response.

Best practice should also refer to the knowledge that health promoters have about what works and does not work in practice including the tools and strategies that have been tested and are accepted as being consistent and effective. Transferring research evidence into practice is not necessarily straightforward because neither the health promoter nor the researchers have the necessary skills to appraise what will work in an outbreak response. The challenges of an evidence-based practice include the poor availability of information and the interpretation of specialist data such as anthropological findings. To improve this situation, it is necessary to broaden what is accepted as an evidence base for health promotion, create better methods for evidence synthesis and differentiate more clearly between theory and what works in practice (Marks 2002).

Health promotion programmes are increasingly expected to justify what they do by providing evidence of their effectiveness. However, what counts as evidence can be a contested issue, partly because it is not always possible to measure the impact, especially interventions to address the broader determinants of health (Rychetnik and Wise 2004). Assessing change can be verified through different methods including a triangulation of information taken from various sources such as programme plans, practitioner logs, minutes of meetings, surveys and activity reports. Triangulation refers to the use of a variety of quantitative and

## BOX 2.1: Informed consent

Informed consent is based upon respect for the dignity and autonomy of every person. A person is fully informed about the benefits and possible risks of an intervention, procedure or treatment as well as the risks of the absence of the procedure or treatment. Informed consent creates a duty for health promoters to provide accurate, understandable and complete information to make the necessary informed decision about participating. Informed consent should help people to make a decision which is in their own interest after the information that is conveyed has been clearly understood (UNAIDS 2007).

qualitative methods; several evaluators, each with differing points of view; or a combination, to make an assessment of the same change (Sechrest 1997).

Secondary sources of data are useful for investigating broader questions in the response and include Demographic and Health Surveys, programme reports and field notes. In some cases, secondary sources might be recent and complete enough so that no additional data collection is required. More commonly, however, gathering the evidence needed to develop or evaluate an intervention requires primary data collection. Primary data collection involves obtaining information directly from the source by using both quantitative and qualitative approaches.

# QUANTITATIVE APPROACHES TO DATA COLLECTION

Quantitative approaches collect data that is in numerical form such as statistics focusing on the rates of morbidity and mortality in a population by using, for example, closed-ended questionnaires and epidemiological sources.

## Epidemiological data

Epidemiological data consist of the patterns, causes, and effects of health and disease conditions in defined populations including statistics, government surveillance data, health surveys and disease registries. These data help policy decisions and evidence-based practice by identifying risk factors for disease and preventive healthcare goals. Epidemiological studies aim to identify causal relationships between exposure to risks and health outcomes and use a range of techniques

---

**BOX 2.2: Early epidemiological techniques and cholera outbreaks**

John Snow (1813–1858) was one of the first people to systematically use epidemiological techniques in London in 1849. He investigated data on cholera mortality by using a new numeric method that revealed the rate was much higher in certain areas which drew its water from heavily polluted sections of the River Thames. His investigations in the Broad Street district were able to show that there was a marked difference in cholera rates when one company moved its water intake source to a less polluted section of the river, whereas another company did not. When another epidemic occurred in 1854, his detailed house-to-house investigation provided conclusive evidence that the water supplied by one company to the Broad Street pump was the source of the cholera. The pump was sealed to stop it from being used by residents and the epidemic slowed down. Legislation in 1857 later required all companies to filter their water supply, and a greater appreciation developed that environmental factors could have an impact on the health of the public (Crosier 2012).

including observational studies and experimental epidemiology that covers randomised control trials, field trials and community trials (Adetunji 2008).

Health profiles are a summary of epidemiological data for a particular population, for example, for a country sub-divided into regions, provinces, towns and communities. Health profiles are usually produced by the government and show how one geographical area compares to the national and regional average. This comparative information then helps to make decisions to prioritise and plan services to address disease outbreaks (Network of Public Health Observatories 2013). Epidemiology has proved effective in establishing the causes of endemic diseases such as malaria but continues to experience difficulty in regard to health issues for which causation is complex such as with immunisation.

> Communities are open to rational discussion and health promoters are well placed to engage with them to offer advice that is based on sound evidence.

## Lay epidemiology

Lay epidemiology describes the processes by which people in their everyday lives interpret risks (Allmark and Tod 2006), including risks to their health. To reach conclusions about risks, people access information from a variety of sources including the mass media, the Internet, friends and family. Lay epidemiology can be an empowering experience for people because it can help them to challenge health professionals in the following ways:

1. People have recognized that some health messages can change. Health messaging that does not tell the whole truth, for example, by exaggerating the risks of a particular behaviour or the benefits of changing that behaviour, can also confuse the situation.
2. People have cultural and personal values that undermine the meaning of health messages; for example, people can choose not to change a behaviour simply because it may be damaging to their health when they believe that the benefits of that behaviour outweigh the risk.
3. People can view any particular health behaviour in at least three ways: (1) It is bad because it is poisonous. (2) It is bad but desirable. (3) It is bad in some ways but good in others. People's perception of risk therefore depends on their circumstances, culture and values and an 'all things considered' approach is taken (Allmark and Tod 2006).

The attempts of those in authority to manipulate the public can place lay epidemiology as a means for communities to validate their concerns and to gain more control over their lives. Lay epidemiology poses a challenge to those in authority because it does not necessarily accept that professional advice is the dominant perspective. Alternatively, information can provide a bridge between

## BOX 2.3: The prevention paradox

The prevention paradox occurs when targeting the behaviour of the majority of the population, who are at a low-to-medium risk, has little effect at the individual level. An overreliance on simple health messaging targeting the majority of the population has led to mistrust in the public, people feel that risk does not apply to them, and they reject the advice (Hunt and Emslie 2001).

those in authority and those in civil society by explaining that the community has a valuable role in the implementation of the programme.

# KNOWLEDGE, ATTITUDE AND PRACTICE SURVEYS

The knowledge, attitude and practice (KAP) approach can be used to promote and evaluate an increase in the knowledge, attitude and practices or behaviours of targeted individuals; groups; and communities. The approach has three key steps: (1) provision of new knowledge, (2) acceptance of and the development of a positive attitude towards the new knowledge, and (3) an intention to take action to a change a related behaviour or practice (Corcoran 2013).

A KAP survey can be designed to provide a representative study of a specific population by collecting information on what is known (knowledge), believed (attitude) and done (practice) in relation to a particular health topic such as hand-washing. KAP surveys typically use a mixed methods approach. They collect data by using a structured, standardized questionnaire and/or use focus group discussions and individual interviews. The data analysis can provide programme managers with the information that they need to select effective interventions (World Health Organization 2008c). Another important role for KAP surveys is to provide essential data for demonstrating the impact of programme activities. This is achieved by measuring the knowledge, attitude and practices of the target population before and then after a specific intervention to demonstrate actual outcomes (Action Against Hunger 2013). A 'before and after study' has no comparison group, and the attributing causality is ascertained by asking people why they had changed their behaviour, by using, for example, a self-reporting questionnaire, a focus group or one-to-one interviews (Jirojwong and Liamputtong 2009).

## Designing a KAP survey

The goal of the sampling design is to interview as few people or households as is necessary, but enough such that the data can be reliably quantified so that it is accurate and representative. For a sample to be representative, it must be large enough and also must be randomly chosen; for example, each household in the target population has an equal chance of being interviewed. For greater accuracy, different types of surveys require different degrees of statistical accuracy, which will require different sample sizes; for example, a KAP survey generally aims for a 10% accuracy.

The design of a KAP survey has six steps:

*Step 1* defines the survey objectives and contains information about how to access existing information, the purpose of the survey and the main areas of enquiry, the survey population and sampling plan.

*Step 2* develops the survey protocol, outlines elements to include in the survey and the key research questions, a work plan and a budget.

*Step 3* designs the survey questionnaire and proposes steps for pre-testing and finalising and for making a data analysis plan.

*Step 4* implements the KAP survey, recruits and trains survey supervisors and interviewers.

*Step 5* analyses the data.

*Step 6* uses the data to translate the survey findings into action, produces the study report and disseminates the survey findings (World Health Organization 2008c).

Systematic sampling can be applied if the given population is logically homogeneous, because systematic sample units are uniformly distributed over the population and therefore the chosen sampling interval should not hide a pattern. For example, if a sample of 8 houses from a community of 120 houses (120/8 = 15) were to be sampled, then every 15th house is chosen after a random starting point between 1 and 15. If the random starting point is 11, then the houses selected are 11, 26, 41, 56, 71, 86, 101 and 116. However, if every 15th house was a corner house then this pattern would threaten the randomness of the sampling of the population. This is random sampling with a system because from the sampling frame, a starting point is chosen at random and choices thereafter are at regular intervals (Action Against Hunger 2013).

## Rapid KAP surveys

KAP surveys can be time-consuming and expensive. In a disease outbreak, new information is required quickly, often daily, to best meet the requirements of rapidly changing circumstances. Rapid KAP surveys are a convenient means to acquire reliable, 'quick and dirty' information in the field. The goal is to gather information quickly but by interviewing as few people or households as possible, providing reliably quantified data in a short time frame.

The Intensified Training for an Ebola Response Project (ITERP) conducted a rapid KAP survey in the western area rural district of Sierra Leone, an area of high transmission between 10 to 16 March 2015. The ITERP was undertaken in three wards – Grafton, Kossoh Town and Jui – occupied by 42,749 people, living in 9406 households. The purpose was to gain insight into community knowledge, attitudes and practices in regard to Ebola control and to identify barriers to the containment of the virus. Public education and social mobilisation campaigns had been met with resistance from communities, people did not report suspected cases and undertook unsafe burial practices. The first step was to involve community leaders to help improve awareness, attitudes and practices. House-to-house interviews were conducted by 30 trained health promoters using a cluster sampling design in 35 villages in Jui (13), Kossoh Town (5) and Grafton (17). Random sampling was used to select 466 households for interviews as follows: (1) Select three or four households in the north, south, east and west of each village. Randomly select the first household in each direction and then choose the next-door neighbour, and so on. Members from at least 12 households were interviewed in each village. (2) Randomly select one eligible family member (between the ages of 20 and 60 years) from each selected household. Approximately, 51% of people interviewed were females, 27.68% were high school students and 55.37% were Muslims. It was found that knowledge about Ebola was high. There was a positive attitude towards prevention, and almost all the participants knew the reporting phone number for suspected cases. Of the participants, 62% had a history of regular travel between urban and rural areas. The implementing agency, contrary to the findings of the rapid KAP survey, concluded that it was a priority to further strengthen public education on the symptoms and modes of transmission (Jiang et al. 2016). The gap between knowledge and practice had not been fully understood by the implementing agency; knowledge about Ebola was already high but supportive practices were low. The solution was not more public education but rather an improvement of the quality of communication through more face-to-face dialogue with people living in areas of high transmission.

## QUALITATIVE APPROACHES TO DATA COLLECTION

Qualitative methods include one-to-one and focus group interviews that draw upon the knowledge and experiences of people affected by the disease outbreak. In qualitative interviewing, the aim is to discover the interviewee's own framework of meanings and to avoid imposing the interviewer's assumptions. The interviewer needs to remain open to the possibility that the variables that emerge may be very different from those that might have been predicted at the outset. The interviewer also needs to be sensitive to the language and concepts used by the interviewee and check that they have understood the meanings of the respondent. The flexibility of the interviewing technique is that it can allow a change in the pace and direction of the interview to avoid any misunderstandings during the inquiry (Britten 1995).

### Qualitative interviewing

There are two main types of qualitative interviewing: unstructured and semi-structured. Unstructured interviews may cover only one or two issues; and although semi-structured interviews are also conducted using an informal structure consisting of open-ended questions that define the area to be explored, the interviewer may diverge to pursue an idea in more detail and depth. The less structured the interview, the less the questions are determined and standardised in advance of the interview. However, most interviews will have a list of core questions that define the areas to be covered. Questions should be open ended, neutral, sensitive and clear to the interviewee, usually starting with questions that the interviewee can easily answer and then proceeding to more difficult and sensitive topics.

## Observational methods

Observational methods have two key components: descriptive and analytical. Descriptive observations pertain to who, what, where and when in regard to a health-related event. Analytical observations deal more with the how of a health-related event. In practice, observational methods involve systematic, detailed observation of behaviour and talk, watching and recording what people do and say. This can involve asking questions and analysing documents, but the primary focus on observation makes it distinct from a qualitative interview (Mays and Pope 1995). 'Observer' as 'participant' is essentially a short interaction with the respondents with no enduring relationship based on lengthy observation. The important advantage of observation is that it can help to overcome the discrepancy between what people say and what they actually do. It circumvents the biases inherent in the accounts people give of their actions caused by factors such as the wish to present themselves in a good light, differences in recall, selectivity and the influences of the roles they occupy. It is impossible to record everything during this process; so, it is inevitably selective and relies on the interviewer to document what he or she observes. Therefore, it is vital that the observations are systematically recorded and analysed (Mays and Pope 1995), and as far as possible the interviewer aims to record exactly what happened.

## Starting the inquiry to collect qualitative information

The initial part of the inquiry uses unstructured interviews with key informants to identify the main theme of the study in the specific cultural context. Unstructured one-to-one interviews are used to discover the interviewee's own framework of meanings. This type of interview dispenses with formal schedules and ordering of questions and relies on the social interaction between the interviewer and the informant to elicit information (Minichiello et al. 1990). The unstructured interview takes on the appearance of a normal everyday conversation. However, it is always a controlled conversation, which is geared to the interviewer's interests. The element of control is minimal but present to keep the informant relating to his or her own experiences that are relevant to the issue (Burgess 1982). More than one unstructured interview can be used so that further questioning can be based on previous interviews. These interviewers should consist mostly of clarification and probing for more depth and detail. It is important to carry out as many unstructured interviews as are necessary to be sure that all the main headings have been identified. The interviewees can be different but the interviews are to be based on the same themes and might begin with the interviewer asking, 'This interview is about (the subject) in your cultural context. Can you tell me about your experiences, what you think this means and how it works in your communities?' The interviews can be held at the interviewees' places of work, homes or in a neutral setting, at a predetermined and convenient time. The interviews are recorded either manually or by using a tape recorder and normally last between 30 and 90 minutes.

## Gaining in-depth information

The findings of the unstructured interviews provide the main headings for the next part of the inquiry, semi-structured group interviews. The questions do not have a fixed order or wording, but act as a guide to the interviewer who uses them in small groups consisting of participants of similar characteristics. The purpose of the interviews is to provide more depth and comprehension to the main headings and anecdotal information to highlight the findings. The selection of participants for the interviews is undertaken to ensure a representative range of age and socioeconomic background of the people in the community. Group interviews are a quick and convenient way to simultaneously collect data. This means that instead of the interviewer asking each person to respond to a question in turn, there is some interaction and people are encouraged to talk, ask questions, exchange anecdotes and to comment on other experiences in the group. Some of the potential advantages are that the technique does not discriminate against people who cannot read or write and encourages participation and discussion, especially from those who might normally feel that they have nothing to say.

When putting together focus groups, it is important to consider the size and, on average, 6–12 people participate in each group because fewer than six participants does not generate a critical mass of interaction and groups larger than 8–10 people can be difficult to give everyone a chance to sufficiently voice their opinions. The group setting can silence individual voices of disagreement and it is these contradictions that the interviewer may want to gain access to as a part of the findings. The presence of other interviewees may also compromise the confidentiality of the session; however, groups are not always inhibiting and may actively facilitate the discussion of sensitive topics.

The success of the group interviews depends on both the skill of the facilitator and the discussion environment. Sessions should be relaxed, in a comfortable and familiar setting, refreshments may be available and the seating should be arranged in a sequence acceptable to the participants. The facilitator should be able to use debate to continue the conversation beyond the stage where it might have otherwise ended. The facilitator should be able to use disagreement to encourage participants to elucidate their point of view and to clarify why they think as they do. Basically, the facilitator should be sensitive to the group and to its particular dynamics (Kitzinger 1995). It should be noted that a limitation of using any participatory technique is that it will require skilled facilitation, and within a programme context this may sometimes not be realistic to achieve because of poor professional competencies.

> ## BOX 2.4: Data saturation
>
> Saturation refers to the point in the qualitative data collection process when all the viewpoints and information about the issue have been voiced already by participants. Saturation occurs when the last two qualitative inquiries, for example, focus group discussions, do not reveal any new insights or ideas that were not mentioned in previous interviews. However, if the discussions are still generating new insights, then more qualitative interviewing sessions may be necessary (Healthcompass 2017).

## Keeping a record of the inquiry

Several different ways can be used by the interviewer to help compile a record of events; for example, a notebook or a laptop can be used to keep detailed records of events, conversations, activities and descriptions. The type of notes can be distinguished as either quick or fully comprehensive recording exactly what is actually said. Mental notes are made of discussions or observations after the event; jotted notes are quick, shorthand notes to remind the interviewer of events. Full field notes are the running notes made throughout the day during or after the observational period and are both descriptive and analytical. The descriptive notes portray the context in which the observations and discussions took place. The analytical notes try to make sense of what has been observed and may be made after the observation when the interviewer has more time to reflect and clarify his or her impressions (Glesne and Peshkin 1992).

## Analysing the qualitative information

The aim of the analysis of the qualitative information is to look both for areas of common ground and differences between the respondents rather than providing a number of separate accounts. There are software packages for qualitative data analysis such as Nvivo that are designed for working with very rich text-based information where deep levels of analysis, often on large volumes of data, are required. The recommended procedure for use in the field is a simpler, cut-and-paste technique which is quick and cost effective for small amounts of qualitative data. The information, which is available in the form of written or printed field notes and transcribed interviews, goes through a process of disaggregation and re-aggregation by using the following steps:

1. The process of disaggregation begins when copies are made of the original field notes. The copies are used to identify a classification system for the major categories of discussion. The categories are identified in the text by using colours to highlight their presence in the text. The recorded text is thoroughly reread and all the marked relevant phrases, sentences or exchanges of recorded conversation are checked.

2. Once the colour coding is complete the marked text is 'cut-up' and sorted into files that have been marked one for each category. The categories will form the headings of the discussion of the findings.
3. The process of re-aggregation happens by rereading each category file to analyse the content in its new context alongside information of a similar nature. New insights and confirmations begin to emerge and the structure of the findings to form.

## Validation in using qualitative information

Validity in using qualitative information can be problematic, for at least three reasons: (1) to an extent, people are assessing their own work; (2) perceptions are prone to recall bias; and (3) the assessment may be influenced by the dynamics of the group, the evaluator or the techniques used (Nutbeam and Bauman 2011).

Guba and Lincoln (1989) suggest the following considerations for a participatory evaluation that can be applied to help maintain rigour, validity and credibility:

- Verification of data with stakeholders, for example, to cross-check cultural interpretations
- Triangulation using different methods and data sources
- A clear documentation of the process from data collection to conclusions
- Verification of interpretations by other evaluators through inter-observer agreement
- Critical self-reflection on meanings of the findings and relevance to stakeholders.

Validity concerns can be further offset by having an emphasis on people providing reasons and examples for their assessments, for example, by providing a brief account of the history and context of the conclusions reached by the individual or group (Bell-Woodard et al. 2005).

> It is essential to have a coordination mechanism to track and to share the findings of all data collection and research that is carried out in the response.

Qualitative investigation techniques do have limitations because they are exploratory in nature to stimulate dialogue, elicit a range of responses and to generate ideas. Because of the limited number of participants, unstructured questioning procedures, and the potential for one respondent's opinions to influence those of others, the findings are not necessarily always considered as being conclusive but rather well-informed guidance.

## COLLECTING QUALITATIVE INFORMATION IN A CROSS-CULTURAL CONTEXT

Health promoters often work with different cultural groups; however, they may not have the ability to speak the local language, hold a different belief and value system, have poor communication and different styles of interaction, attitudes towards time and political sensitivities. It is recognised that knowledge of the local language, although important, is not essential and that building a rapport with potential participants is more a function of time spent on site and of interpersonal skills than it is of cultural identity and linguistics (Ginsberg 1988). In practice, it may not be possible to have a facilitated group discussion due to the language and cultural differences between the health promoter and participants. In this case a facilitated design can be used that takes the cultural context into account. This requires a facilitator to be appointed to work with the health promoter, one who is familiar with the cultural context. Facilitation introduces higher levels of control, the ability to focus on specific goals within a limited time period and is not merely translation or interpretation. Apart from accurate interpretation to the health promoter during the course of the meeting, the ways in which facilitators work in the group setting such as their role, style, background and appearance are crucial in shaping interactions.

Cross-cultural facilitators are able to speak the local language, understand local customs and more easily explain complex concepts without the need for translation, and this will help to expedite the meeting. However, in a non-westernised context, facilitators tend to lead the discussion and take a directive rather than a participatory approach and encourage discussion but do not try to involve all the participants. The facilitator can dominate and direct group interaction and not allow the focus of discussion to move towards its members (Laverack and Brown 2003) and must therefore be carefully supervised.

> Good facilitation is crucial to collecting information but can be hard to find and must be constantly monitored for quality of delivery.

Possessing the necessary skills for facilitation does not guarantee against bias, but proper training may reduce unintentional influences. Although high rapport is always the goal of skilful facilitation, in a cross-cultural context this may have to be achieved through roles embodying lower levels of rapport and differing levels of engagement. The purpose of this approach is to better position the facilitators to achieve an empathetic understanding of the participants. The facilitators may have to be prepared to be more and less directive and engaged when collecting qualitative information, adapting their approach to the specific requirements of the participants. This can be described as an 'inward' and 'outward' movement by the facilitators towards a terrain of empathy (Glesne and Peshkin 1992). A key feature, and therefore a key skill, is the ability of the facilitator to understand the perspective of the people that they are facilitating. Other skills are tolerance for ambiguity, adaptiveness, capacity for tacit learning, courtesy and respect (Seefeldt 1985). Appropriate tools for collecting cross-cultural information include case studies and interviews which use a strong narrative and the oral traditions of different cultures. The approach should use both qualitative and quantitative information to triangulate the findings. The tools should also be flexible in the time frame, be participatory and use culturally sensitive questioning.

## DATA COLLECTION THAT PROMOTES PARTICIPATION

In practice, the participation of the community in data collection will be through 'selective representation', for example, of elected individuals taking part in a focus group meeting. However, care must be taken to avoid this becoming empty and frustrating for those who are not directly involved and that in effect may allow those in authority to claim that all sides were considered while only a few benefited. There are a range of participatory methodologies that actively involve people in the gathering of information, for example, participatory rapid appraisal techniques. The advantages of using a participatory approach over conventional assessments include the following: (1) it is self-educative, (2) it is self-improving, (3) it enables stakeholders to monitor progress, and (4) it builds upon and improves skills (Mays and Pope 1995). It should be noted that the limitations of using participatory techniques is that they require skilled facilitation, that may not be available in an outbreak context because of a lack of professional competence, and because the gender or culture of the facilitator influence the responses of the participants.

In a practical sense, the participatory approach should be based on the shared experiences of the participants which, as far as possible, are not influenced by the methodology or have not been biased by the person collecting the data. However, their presence can directly influence the findings, even at its most basic; for example, having someone observing actions may affect the validity of information by stimulating modifications in behaviour or self-questioning among those participating (Mays and Pope 1995). The participants themselves may also be a source of 'subject bias'; for example, participants, knowing the importance or reward they will receive from a good result or the result desired will change their behaviour during data collection.

Participatory rapid or rural appraisal (PRA) is an approach that aims to incorporate the knowledge and opinions of local people in the planning, evaluation and management of programmes. PRA enables people to collect, share and analyse information that they themselves have identified as being important. It is not a single technique but a collection of participatory and non-participatory approaches and methods. PRA has also been used for its potential to help empower communities on the basis that it actively involves the marginalized, assesses their needs, builds capacities and includes them in decision-making processes. The large range of techniques that have been developed for its implementation can be divided into four categories: (1) group dynamics such as learning contracts, role reversals, feedback sessions; (2) sampling such as transect walks, wealth ranking, social mapping; (3) interviewing such as focus group discussions, semi-structured interviews, triangulation; and (4) visualization such as diagrams, matrix scoring and timelines (Chambers 1997).

> Participatory data collection that does not offer people the means to transform information into action is not empowering.

To ensure that people are not excluded from the participatory process the PRA largely uses oral and visual communication techniques such as pictures, physical objects and stories. Although PRA can produce a large amount of information, it does not always offer a means to transform this into action, a crucial stage that promotes empowerment. Validity in using participatory techniques can also be problematic because personal perceptions are prone to recall bias or the assessment may be influenced by the dynamics of the group, the evaluator or the techniques used (Nutbeam and Bauman 2011). A new paradigm of professionalism has therefore emerged in the use of PRA techniques in which the key focus is on decentralisation and empowerment. Decentralisation means that resources and discretion are devolved to the participants. Empowerment means that people are enabled to take more control over their lives, and secure ownership and the control of their assets (Chambers 1997). The inclusion of PRA techniques in large-scale programmes in which the agenda becomes externally driven rather than community driven runs the real risk of becoming simply a needs assessment rather than a participatory and empowering experience.

## THE ROLE OF ANTHROPOLOGY

> Anthropological insights can significantly contribute to the disease outbreak response because they help us to understand the complexity of the problem.

Anthropological studies usually require an in-depth and sometimes a long-term input, whereas in an outbreak response, new information is required quickly as the situation changes, often on a daily basis. As the response progresses, it is rapidly obtained information, produced by epidemiologists and social scientists, which can best meet the requirements of the changing circumstances. Anthropology is considered to be a 'slow science' in which evidence is collected in a steady and methodical way over an extended period of time. Anthropologists are trained to provide in-depth accounts which can be difficult to translate into practical recommendations, compounded by a poor understanding of how programmes function. Anthropological recommendations are sometimes disregarded for being too vague; as a consequence, these valuable insights may not be widely used in the response. The missing link has been a discussion between the programme manager and the anthropologist. This would be best performed with an intermediary person, one with the skills to provide an interpretation of the practical relevance of the anthropological findings.

## Anthropological recommendations for response actions

In the West African Ebola response, anthropologists were able to provide significant insights into complex cultural practices regarding death and burial. For example, the belief that the dead can be aggravated if their last words are not heard and honoured, if they are buried outside of the village to wander eternally rather than being with their family (or be returned to it as a stone from the tomb) or if the correct sacrifices are not made. It was also important to understand that special cultural rules and protocols have to be followed for burial rights such as for pregnant women, uninitiated girls, babies and prominent men in the community (Fairhead 2014). However, the style of anthropological information presented was often rich, dense and in a narrative form that can be difficult to interpret, especially in the context of specific operational requirements. The responsibility to interpret this information into relevant response actions has traditionally been with the programme manager. These professionals, no matter how highly skilled, often lack the skills to quickly interpret anthropological information; consequently, it can be disregarded. Anthropologists sometimes do provide recommendations in an outbreak response, but the relevance is not clear to what needs to happen in a programme context.

One solution is not to use anthropological information but to rely on rapid assessment techniques that can be more easily translated into recommendations. However, it is still important that anthropological information is used in the response and that the format of the information is relevant to the needs of programme managers. Anthropological reports should include a set of concise and relevant recommendations that are categorised for each activity, for example, for an Ebola response, in regard to the following:

1. *Case finding and contact tracing*: extended family structure, communication, reasons for high or low contact tracing
2. *Case management*: low patronage of community care centres, health-seeking behaviour, the reasons for fear and stigma
3. *Safe and dignified burials*: unsafe burial practices and alternative customs, reasons for unknown transmission, community perceptions
4. *Community engagement*: reasons for community resistance, gender representation, survivor needs, fears and stigmas

The recommendations provided should be in order of priority, and it is important that they are not presented as an abbreviated list of research findings but must be relevant and realistic to the programme delivery. The anthropologist may wish to discuss the draft recommendations with a programme manager before submitting the report. Some examples of recommendations are provided below:

- Ensure an epidemiologist collaborates with the anthropologist to enhance understanding and interpretation of sociocultural determinants of EVD.
- Recruit more women in the (programme name) response teams because they are more likely to be responsive to the needs of other women and accepted by other women.

- A review of the effectiveness of the Community Watch Committees approach in Guinea should be carried out as soon as is practicable and the results presented to the relevant agency.
- Survivor networks and support groups (programme name) should continue to be assisted.

The implementing agency must ensure that the recommendations are discussed in person with the relevant programme manager after submission, including any constraints for delivery and any support that may be required. If the recommendations are directly used in the response the anthropologist should be informed about how his or her work has had an influence on the disease outbreak.

## Understanding complex cultural situations

Understanding complex cultural situations and how they apply to everyday procedures in a disease outbreak is crucial to the success of a response. Communities are willing to work with health promoters to identify solutions that can satisfy complex cultural needs and protect against disease transmission. In Sierra Leone, for example, the family a pregnant woman who had died of Ebola had requested the response team to remove the foetus so that the mother and baby could be buried separately. The cultural belief is that when a pregnant woman dies, the child should be removed and buried separately. Otherwise, there is a 'fault' and the order of things is disrupted. The response team considered extracting the foetus to be too dangerous because of cross-contamination. Eventually, an agreement was reached that the woman could be buried without extracting the foetus, but that a reparation ritual with various offerings and ceremonies would need to be conducted. The response team agreed to pay for the reparation ritual, and the burial finally took place (Fairhead 2014). The delay of the burial of the pregnant woman and the anxiety caused to her family could have been avoided if a proper understanding of the situation had quickly been effectively communicated to the programme manager.

Anthropological information can also be used to develop training exercises for programme staff to better understand the sensitive cultural context in which they are working. For example, the box below uses an exercise to explore understandings of a safe and dignified burial in the community.

> Respect for the local culture and a recognition of community autonomy to plan and implement their own actions is crucial to the success of a response.

Understanding complex cultural situations can provide useful information throughout the progression of an outbreak and requires specific skills to collect, interpret and then to translate the information into clear programmatic recommendations. This can be a combination of qualitative, quantitative or rapid data collection techniques depending on the stage of progression and the urgency of the needs of the response. For example, the box below uses an exercise to explore understandings of a safe and dignified burial in the community.

---

## BOX 2.5: Burial role play

The purpose of this exercise is to help explore understandings of what a typical burial in the community would entail, including the funeral and safe and dignified burial protocols and who is involved at each step. Practical solutions can be identified about what can be done if burial services are unsafe or culturally insensitive. The exercise would normally take about 1 hour.

Begin by reminding community members that you are an outsider and that you are keen to learn about the specific practices in the community related to funerals and burials. Ask community members if they could act out a typical burial by using role play, or if this does not feel comfortable they could describe it. Use the role play/description to ask questions related to burial procedures in the community; for example, if someone from this community is sick, where is the best place for them to die? If a death happens in the 'bush' or outside the village, what will happen? What if a death happens away from home and a body cannot be brought back? What should be done? Are there any special procedures for certain types of deaths (e.g. prominent person, first born, pregnant women, uninitiated girls)? If funeral/burial cannot be done properly, how can a 'fault' be repaired? How are debts settled after death? How is property and inheritance settled?

Use the safe and dignified burial protocol to describe what is happening at each step. Do not immediately describe the steps yourself; allow community members to look at the pictures or images and then discuss. After they have had some time to discuss, you may answer any questions they have or clarify any points that were not clear. Discuss whether the steps are suitable and appropriate for this community. Can people accept these burials? If not, what modifications are needed? How do the burials fit within existing local protocols? Encourage discussion and debate on these different issues and do not interrupt if discussion becomes heated. There will likely be very strong feelings about this topic, and it may be particularly sensitive if there have been recent deaths in the community. Allow community members the chance to accept or reject the protocol. If they reject them, find out why and what could be done to make them more acceptable (SMAC 2014).

# 3

# The public communication approach

---

> **KEY POINTS**
>
> - Disease outbreak responses are controlled by agencies that use top-down approaches to change people's behaviours rather than giving them more control over their lives.
> - Improving knowledge does not guarantee a desirable change in people's behaviour.
> - The technical language that the health promoter chooses to use will determine the nature of the professional relationship with other people.
> - The use of Information and Communication Technology is rapidly changing the way in which people are mobilised and communicate with one another in disease outbreaks.
> - Knowledge, attitude and practice surveys show that the levels of awareness are often already high in the general population.

Public communication is an exchange of information among individuals, groups and agencies through various channels such as the mass media, print materials and face-to-face interaction. To be able to communicate effectively requires a systematic approach that includes accurate messaging, a team approach, resources and a strategic plan that creates a dialogue and builds capacity. The communication approach uses language the public understands and that actively engages with people in their everyday lives. Communication can enable people to gain more control over their lives and to make informed choices about a disease outbreak. Risk communication is an interactive exchange of information specifically about the nature of a risk, to address concerns to messages or to legal and institutional arrangements and is discussed separately in Chapter 4.

## EMPOWERMENT OR BEHAVIOUR CHANGE?

The difference between delivering a communication approach that empowers others compared to simply changing their behaviour is in the selection of the strategy. If the strategy gives the health promoter the authority to control the situation, for example, through setting the agenda or releasing specific resources, it is less likely to be empowering. If it facilitates a process of needs assessment, planning and capacity building towards political action by their partners, it has a much better chance of being empowering. The key question for health promoters is, Do I want to help others to empower themselves or to only change their behaviour?

> Disease outbreak responses are controlled by agencies that use top-down approaches to change people's behaviours rather than giving them more control over their lives.

The behaviour change approach can be overly paternalistic and may disregard the individual's own perception of what is important. The behaviour change approach can lead to victim blaming and stigmatisation and to increased inequalities in health, as its focus is on individual behaviours instead of the broader determinants of health. The empowerment approach can lead to helping some groups over other groups. The focus is not primarily on health, and empowered people might still choose to behave in ways that risk damaging their health. However, the empowerment approach, on the whole, is considered to be superior to the behaviour change approach (Tengland 2013) based on moral grounds and increased sustainability.

Both the top-down and bottom-up approaches aim to achieve improvements in health. However, the advantage of empowerment is that it strengthens the autonomy and skills of individuals, groups and communities to achieve better, healthier and more sustainable lives. Behaviour changes do sometimes lead to greater autonomy and control, but this is usually as a secondary effect, such as increased feelings of self-esteem. The solution therefore is to avoid a focus solely on behaviour change and to aim for the attainment of greater autonomous choice and empowerment.

## THE LINK BETWEEN EDUCATION AND EMPOWERMENT

The link between education and empowerment involves more than simply acquiring new information. Knowledge can actually lead to a greater sense of disempowerment when a person is unable to use the new information that they have acquired to improve their circumstances. For example, the message 'regularly wash your hands with soap to avoid cholera' is pointless if the person does not have access to soap, disinfectant or extra water. The link relates to critical education in which the central premise is that education is not neutral but is influenced by the context of one's life. Critical education can be described as the ability to reflect on the assumptions underlying our actions and to contemplate better ways of living (Goodman et al. 1998). Groups cannot intentionally empower themselves without having an understanding of the underlying causes of their powerlessness. This may occur from within the group and can be facilitated through a process that promotes discussion, reflection and action. Increasing critical awareness involves people developing realistic actions to begin to resolve the conditions that have created their powerlessness in the first place. A group dialogue approach can be used to share ideas and experiences and to promote critical thinking by posing problems to allow people to uncover the root causes of their powerlessness.

A key consideration when working with adolescents is the age at which they begin to understand their world in a concrete and abstract way such that they can fully engage with critical education. An approach based on their right to participate as social actors accepts that they act on the world around them. Health promoters can then engage with them about their worlds and involve them in identifying their needs and in decision-making processes. Although there is not a definitive youngest age at which adolescents can be engaged to empower themselves, a guide of 14 years, give or take a year, depending on the individual and the sociocultural context, can be used as a guide in health promotion approaches (Laverack 2013).

## BEHAVIOUR CHANGE COMMUNICATION

A health behaviour is 'an activity undertaken by an individual, regardless of actual or perceived health status, for the purpose of promoting, protecting or maintaining health (World Health Organization 1998, 8). Behaviour change is the process of enabling others to achieve this action. The behavioural approach has been central to health promotion campaigns and focusses on providing people with the knowledge and skills to help them to adopt a healthier lifestyle. A behaviour change approach also recognises the importance of influencing perceived norms and social networks through, for example, family, friends and peer groups.

Behaviour change communication (BCC) is an intervention to promote positive health behaviours that are appropriate to people's settings and is therefore target specific and systematically considers the following in its design: the vulnerability/risk factor of the target group, the conflict and obstacles in the way to the desired change in behaviour, the type of message and communication media which can best reach the target group, the type of resources available, and assessment of existing knowledge of the target group about the issue (UNDP 2002). Social and behaviour change communication is a contemporary adaptation of BCC. This approach identifies behavioural pathways and then uses communication strategies including digital media, broadcast media, community mobilisation, interpersonal communication and advocacy to influence social norms as well as individual behaviours (Center for Communication Programs 2014).

The foundation for BCC is based on the assumption that before individuals and communities can change their behaviours, they must first understand basic facts about a health issue, adopt key attitudes and learn a set of skills. They must also perceive their environment as supporting the change in and the maintenance of their behaviour, such as seeking appropriate treatment, care and support. This process has been identified as having several key steps centred around the provision and acceptance of new information and skills including pre-knowledge, becoming more knowledgeable, having a positive attitude towards the new knowledge, intending to take action to change behaviour, practicing and advocating the behaviour (Corcoran 2013).

## Addressing the gap between knowledge and behaviour change

Communication strategies to promote a change in knowledge and behaviour change have mainly relied upon messages that are delivered to the target population by using mass media techniques. This may have resulted in a difference between knowledge levels and observed or reported behaviour changes. For example, the knowledge of school pupils about the proper use of latrines (98%), safe water supplies (98%) and the prevention of worm infection (95%) was found to be very high in one study covering four provinces in Vietnam (Trinh et al. 1999). However, a study of intestinal worm infection in adults and children (felt to be a reliable indicator of hygiene practice and sanitary conditions) found high rates for roundworm, threadworm and hookworm to be 83%, 94% and 59%, respectively (Needham et al. 1998). Although knowledge about hygiene was high the high level of intestinal worm infection indicates that people were not putting into practice, or able to practice, this knowledge.

Several causes have been identified for the gap between knowledge and behaviour change (UNICEF 2001) including:

- The reliance on a top-down apparatus using didactic, one-directional styles of communication.
- Communication interventions have lacked adequate research.
- There has been poor coordination of communication activities between agencies and sectors.
- Proper audience segmentation has not always been included in programme design, resulting in inappropriate message content and social exclusion of specific groups.
- The demand generated by communication messages has not always been matched by supply.
- Materials development and distribution have not been given sufficient attention.

Another key cause of the gap between knowledge and practice has been weak message content. Public awareness in regard to the Ebola virus disease was high in Liberia, West Africa, but this did not change people's behaviours.

They informed through the mass media to put aside tradition and culture and to 'do the right thing' by following the advice on clinical procedures for safe burials and quarantines. This actually reinforced local perceptions that traditional beliefs and behaviours were barriers to be overcome by the authorities and resulted in people doing the opposite behaviour. Building a narrative of trust through communication is difficult, and community confidence is best strengthened through bottom-up approaches that respect local perspectives (Laverack and Manoncourt 2015). A lack of trust in the system, for example, fear about losing income and of becoming unable to care for sick family members, and a continued threat of becoming infected, can be a cause of denial and community resistance (ACAPS 2015).

The assumption that by improving knowledge an intervention will automatically lead to a change in a person's attitudes and practices is overly simplistic and places too much emphasis on individual responsibility. It is a top-down perspective that people are free to choose healthier options when in fact other factors that determine their health may be out of their control, for example, being unemployed or living in stressful conditions (Holland 2007). The gap between knowledge and behaviour change can be prevented by using a two-way communication between the recipient and a 'significant other' source of information, for example, a family member or a health professional. A two-way communication creates a dialogue in which barriers to resolving health problems can be identified and actions to address the issue can be planned.

> Improving knowledge does not guarantee a desirable change in people's behaviour.

## Message development

The development of effective messaging is core to behaviour change communication and depends on an understanding of the audience. Formative research is the basis for developing effective communication strategies by using a range of quantitative and qualitative methods depending on what information is required to develop, test, and refine messages. The use of quantitative and qualitative data collection is discussed in detail in Chapter 2. This process should be conducted at the beginning of the intervention and is used to gain insight into the health issue or behaviour, the audiences and the main drivers of behaviour that are culturally appropriate. In setting the objectives for the formative research, it is important to consider the information needs to make the necessary decisions. For example, which products and services are required? What are current practices? What is the target population's prior experience with disease? What economic resources are available to the target audience? What products or services are currently available at the household level to address the outbreak? In the context of a disease outbreak, draft messages can be used to more rapidly test and develop the communication materials. Examples of draft messages are provided in Chapter 8 for Zika and yellow fever campaigns. The messages should be continuously refined and adapted as the outbreak develops, although the essential factual information can be delivered at the beginning of the response.

The communication strategy identifies the tools, training materials, message content and images, channels of communication and approach. These may have to be field tested to validate the communication strategy. The result of knowledge, attitude and practice (KAP) surveys or data collection can be used to select the tools and to develop the specific message content. Examples of messages developed for disease outbreaks by using formative research are provided in Chapters 7 and 8. The testing can be achieved through a discussion with the health promoters that will use the strategy and with a selection of the target audience to ensure that it is understandable, culturally appropriate and motivating. Once the draft materials, such as leaflets, and message content have been validated, they can then be produced and distributed and training can be provided for their implementation.

## COMMUNICATION FOR DEVELOPMENT

The World Congress on Communication for Development developed the following definition: 'a social process based on dialogue using a broad range of tools and methods. It is also about seeking change at different levels including listening, building trust, sharing knowledge and skills, building policies, debating and learning for sustained and meaningful change' (World Congress on Communication for Development 2007, 1).

Communication for Development (C4D) gives a voice to communities and provides them with the skills they need to advocate effectively for change. Social and behavioural data are used to plan, implement and evaluate communication initiatives that help increase knowledge, shift attitudes and facilitate positive behaviour change around issues that affect health. The participation of all stakeholders throughout the C4D process allows for local and cultural perspectives to be included in the design, testing and implementation of communication strategies. It creates awareness of people's own rights and changes policy by working with national governments, civil society organizations and development agencies. Championed by United Nations Children's Fund (UNICEF), C4D uses a mix of advocacy, social mobilization and behaviour and social change strategies including in polio eradication and the prevention of HIV/AIDS.

Advocacy involves people acting on behalf of themselves or on behalf of others to argue a position and to influence the outcome of decisions. In health promotion practice advocacy, initiatives are usually started to support particular causes, interest groups and ideologies (Smithies and Webster 1998). Advocacy is an adaptive process of gathering, organizing and formulating information into argument, which is then communicated to others. UNICEF, for example, advocates to influence policy makers, political and social leaders, to create an enabling environment that creates and sustains social transformation.

Social mobilization is a process that engages and motivates a wide range of partners at national and local levels to raise awareness and to create a demand for change. The different stakeholders include community networks, civic groups and faith-based groups that work in a coordinated way to engage with specific populations with planned communication messages.

Behaviour and social change is a consultative process for addressing knowledge, attitudes and practices. It provides relevant information using a mix of media channels and participatory methods. Behaviour change strategies focus on the individual as a locus of change. Socially, it focuses on the community as the unit of change. For behaviours to change, cultural practices, societal norms and structural inequalities have to be changed.

> Knowledge, attitude and practice surveys often show that the levels of awareness are often already high in the general population.

During the Ebola outbreak in West Africa, each of the three affected countries used a different variation on the C4D approach. Liberia applied the principles of C4D, social behaviour change communication and information, education and communication techniques. Sierra Leone also used C4D, with a mixed-methods approach, strong on messaging and print materials. Guinea was the exception: it relied on the use of radio and the Community Watch Committees or 'comité de veille', a community-based approach that in practice did not deliver what was expected. However, the establishment and scale-up of more than 2000 Community Watch Committees throughout Guinea strained monitoring and supervision by both the government and its implementing partners. One estimation suggested that only 25% of the Community Watch Committees were functional and that guidance on community representation was not always respected by local leaders. As the outbreak progressed, the response was slow to adapt to engage people in a dialogue to address deep-seated practices, in particular, those that continued to allow the transmission of the disease such as unsafe burial

## BOX 3.1: Communication for development in West Africa

The findings from the knowledge, attitude and practice (KAP) surveys in Liberia and Sierra Leone during the Ebola outbreak showed that knowledge levels were consistently high, often above 90%. This is an endorsement of the Communication for Development approach used in the response: a combination of mass media, print materials and face-to-face communication. The mass media approach was successful in reaching a large number of households to raise awareness; however, the quality and coverage of the interpersonal communication were variable and were sometimes carried out without sufficient discussion of the key concerns in regard to the spread of the disease (Laverack and Manoncourt 2015).

practices. The outbreak persisted because the response did not use bottom-up approaches quickly enough, did not build a dialogue or promote self-management or failed to convince communities to change their traditional practices (Laverack and Manoncourt 2015). There was also a reliance on hygiene promotion because some agencies did not adapt their messaging to reflect the specific nature of the transmission of the Ebola virus disease.

## SOCIAL MARKETING

Social marketing reflects commercial sector approaches applied to social and health problems that are then resolved by behaviour change (Andreasen 1995). Social marketing has been used in a variety of projects, for example, to eliminate leprosy, increase adherence to medication to treat tuberculosis and to promote immunisation. Social marketing strategies are concerned first with the needs, preferences and social and economic circumstances of the target audience. This information is used to ensure that the most attractive benefits of a product, service or message are offered and that any barriers to its acceptance are addressed (Maibach et al. 2002). Communicating with the target audience about the relative advantages of what is offered is one element of social marketing, as are efforts to address the economic and regulatory environment. The target audience is a specific group of people at which a health-promoting message or product is directed and is identified by several factors including age, gender, level of risk and marital status (Kotler 2000).

Social marketing interventions usually incorporate all or at least a mix of the following '4 P's:

1. Create an enticing 'product' (i.e. the package of benefits associated with the desired action)
2. Minimize the 'price' the target audience believes it must pay in the exchange
3. Make the exchange and its opportunities available in a 'place' that reaches the audience and fits its lifestyles
4. 'Promote' the exchange opportunity with creativity and through channels and tactics that maximise desired responses

Social marketing can be manipulative and does not address underlying environmental and social causes of poor health. Social marketing requires considerable planning, expertise and resources and may therefore not be appropriate in disease outbreaks. However, success has been achieved by adapting social marketing interventions to fit national- or local-level requirements by targeting cultural preferences (Grier and Bryant 2005).

## COMMUNITY RADIO

Radio is often a primary source of information used during disease outbreaks. It is accessible to many communities, transcends literacy barriers and can use local languages. Community radio is a system that provides equipment, training and airtime on local channels, encouraging participation in the media, and it has been used by health promoters to focus on local as well as international issues relevant to a disease outbreak.

---

**BOX 3.2: Community radio and polio in Chad**

Community radio stations were developed to provide a variety of edutainment activities to be broadcast as part of an initiative to eradicate polio in Chad. Radio remains one of the main sources of information that can reach people on immunisation messaging. During the national campaign, 23% of parents in Chad were informed about vaccination through community radio. Almost 40 radio stations disseminated awareness messages and produced edutainment activities in local communities. This was supported by a network of social mobilisers which included 3500 public announcers and 3300 community volunteers. Training workshops were also periodically held to provide better skills in the design and production of public radio programmes, to directly engage communities and to educate them on the importance of vaccination (Maes 2014).

---

Community radio can provide a range of options including talk and entertainment shows to promote the messages in a culturally acceptable way and 'call-in' formats where the public can ask questions on air to a qualified health expert. Radio also offers the space for a debate on issues related to the disease outbreak such as rumours that may not be available in the mass media. Print materials include posters, leaflets, booklets and flip charts and can be used as a part of one-to-one communication to assist the transfer of information working with both literate and non-literate people in conjunction with specific radio broadcasts.

---

**BOX 3.3: Community radio and Ebola in Guinea**

A negative impact of the Ebola outbreak in Guinea was that children did not go to school because schools were not reopened after the summer recess to help prevent the spread of the disease. This affected 1.6 million pupils. To help children catch up on their missed lessons the Ministry of Education worked with a local non-government organisation to develop an emergency community radio programme for a month-long pilot project in Forécariah. The programme was extended to four more districts chosen because they had a low level of school attendance and a high level of Ebola cases. The broadcasts also included a segment about Ebola; how to treat it, how to prevent its spread and the need for good hygiene and hand-washing with soap. It was estimated that the pilot project reached more than 30,000 children and 329 schools in the Forécariah district alone and at least the same number of out-of-school children (UNICEF 2016d).

# SOCIAL MEDIA

The social media refers to technologies which are intended to reach a large audience via mass communication including radio, television, the Internet and mobile phones. Social media also offers an effective channel to target specific population groups at a low cost. For example, during the 2009–2010 H1N1 outbreak and seasonal flu outbreak, the Centers of Disease Control and Prevention and the American government worked together to create social media tools that provided the public with credible, science-based information. This was intended to encourage participation and to communicate messages to influence positive decisions about preventing the H1N1 outbreak and seasonal flu (CDC 2012).

> The use of information and communication technology is rapidly changing the way in which people are mobilised and communicate with one another in disease outbreaks.

The use of information and communication technology (ICT) is rapidly changing the way in which people are able to be mobilised through the growth of social networks such as Facebook. Given the growth in ICT access and use, it is important for agencies to understand and consider how these tools, if used appropriately and with proper planning, monitoring and evaluation, can increase impact, lower costs and expand audience reach. In particular, the use of the short message service (SMS) can be a reliable way to transfer messages to a wide audience. The findings of one study suggest that the use of SMS text messaging is a very effective means of communication for exchange between the pubic and health promoters (Avery-Gomez 2008).

## BOX 3.4: The 'Let's Get Ready!' social media initiative

The 'Let's Get Ready!' social media initiative helped families in China prepare for emergencies by using a 3G mobile website, a mobile application and videos. It was designed to create an interactive and engaging learning experience for children aged 3–6 years and their caregivers. Let's Get Ready! distributed materials on emergency response and preparedness to more than 120,000 children in 15 provinces, and this showed that 68% of families who used the mobile content had taken action, for example, assembled an emergency kit, in preparing for an emergency in their area (Stewart 2013).

The SMS is the most widely used data application internationally because the essential element is not high technology, but universality. Mobile telephones can extend participation, monitoring and transparency, decentralise networks and provide opportunities for local innovation in regard to disease outbreaks. However, they can also be a means by which rumours are spread quickly in the population.

> **BOX 3.5: A cholera outbreak and mobile phones in Tanzania**
>
> In response to an outbreak of cholera among Burundians in a refugee camp in Tanzania, health workers were able to track and monitor new cases through mobile phone technology. The high number of refugees and limited access to drinking water and inadequate sanitation led to an outbreak of nearly 170 cholera cases. It became essential to quickly identify and track cases in real time by using 'RapidPro' technology on mobile phones to allow health workers to quickly notify the authorities of new cases and to report on the progress of each hospitalised case. The mobile phone technology assisted in raising awareness and to geo-locate specific cholera cases, and with other measures such as the provision of safe drinking water and vaccination helped to contain the spread of the disease (Doctors Without Borders 2015; Luthi 2015).

## FACE-TO-FACE COMMUNICATION

Face-to-face communication is individually focussed on a one-to-one (the health promoter to the person) basis and allows a dialogue to develop. This is based on a sharing of knowledge and experiences in a two-way communication that is necessary to help individuals to better retain information, clarify personal issues and develop skills. An example of using face-to-face communication is helping a person to understand how certain cultural practices can cause the transmission of a disease.

Technical terms are a part of the everyday language of health promoters. However, the use of specialist language is often confusing both to lay people and to other health workers not part of their professional sub-culture. This can contribute to a sense of powerlessness by showing a lack of access to knowledge and the expert power of the person using the language. It is important for health promoters to understand the influence of their language and to be sensitive to the position and perceptions of others. Such awareness is termed a 'reflexive practice' in which health promoters are critical about the way they use their knowledge to have an influence over others.

> The technical language that the health promoter chooses to use will determine the nature of their professional relationship with other people.

To improve face-to-face communication the health promoter can follow a simple procedure of listening, giving advice and obtaining and providing feedback to others. Listening is an active process focusing on what the individual is saying and, if necessary, helping the speaker to express his or her feelings or to give an opinion on an issue. When giving advice the health promoter is exerting his or her expert power to persuade someone into actually accepting a subservient role.

The relationship grants the health promoter the right to prescribe advice while the other person accepts an obligation to comply with the advice. This is sometimes a necessary communication style when, for example, giving a precise instruction about the self-administration of a medicine by the patient to ensure his or her compliance. Obtaining and giving feedback enables the health promoter to clarify what the person wants and ensures they have understood previous communication messages or have retained skills. This can be facilitated by using closed questions that require short factual (yes or no) answers or it can be based on an open form of questioning to provide fuller answers. Giving feedback reinforces the strengths of the person's knowledge level and encourages the sharing of concerns, feelings and opinions, but the discussion should be guided by the health promoter.

## Peer education

Peer education helps people to promote health-enhancing changes among their peers. Rather than health professionals educating members of the public, lay persons are felt to be in the best position to encourage healthy behaviour in each other (Kelly et al. 1992). Peer education is usually initiated by health promoters who recruit members of the target audience, typically about the same age, to serve as educators. The recruited peer educators are trained in relevant health information and communication skills and then engage their peers in conversations about the issue of concern, seeking to promote health-enhancing behaviour change. The intention is that familiar people, giving locally relevant and meaningful suggestions, in a local language and taking account of the local context, will be more likely to promote health. They may work alongside the health promoter, run educational activities on their own or actually take the lead in organizing and implementing activities. Youth peer educators have shown in some cases to be more effective than adults in establishing norms and in changing attitudes, for example, related to sexual behaviour change (UNICEF 2013). Peer education has also been popular in HIV prevention, especially involving young people, sex workers and intravenous drug users. Despite its popularity, the evidence about peer education is mixed, seemingly working in some contexts but not in others. One study comparing peer education among sex workers in India and South Africa, for example, found that the more successful Indian group benefited from a supportive social and political context, and a more effective community development ethos, rather than the biomedical focus of the South African intervention (Cornish and Campbell 2009).

Befriending is a variation of peer education that offers supportive, reliable one-to-one relationships through peers with people who would otherwise be socially isolated. It is an internationally recognised approach that offers voluntary support for young people, families, people with disabilities and older people. The results of befriending can be very significant and often provides people with a new direction in life, opening up a range of activities and leads to increased self-confidence. However, both befriending and peer education interventions can have a high attrition rate as volunteers may leave the programme because of personal and financial constraints (Falkirk Council/HealthProm 2013).

---

**BOX 3.6: My Future Is My Choice – Life skills programme through peer education**

The most successful interventions to control the spread of HIV have been the availability of antiretroviral drugs, peer education and out-reach activities. To counter the growing threat of HIV to young people in Namibia, 'My Future is My Choice' was designed to reach them, through other young people, with sexual health information. Young people between the ages of 14 and 21 years received training to provide information and life skills specifically for HIV/AIDS prevention, substance abuse and rape. Each peer educator developed an action plan to reach at least 10 friends and/or become a member of an AIDS drama, role play or debating club. The peer educators used games to teach skills in a fun way, small group work and discussion time for young people as this helped them to think more critically about their personal circumstances. Young people provided the day-to-day management and supervision of the life skills programme and training, distributed materials and con-doms and collaborated with schools and clinics. The young people who went through the programme had a positive change in attitude towards, and learned new skills in, condom use. A major constraint of the pro-gramme was sustaining the involvement of the young peer educators through the correct level of incentives. The issue of using incentives when working with volunteers is discussed in Chapter 4. An enabling environment was also necessary through the involvement of parents, teachers, local leaders and service providers (UNICEF 2016e).

---

Peer education should be seen as a strategy that can be used alongside other health promotion approaches; for example, it has been used effectively to comple-ment skills-based health education on condom promotion and youth-friendly health services (UNICEF 2013).

## USING A STORYTELLING APPROACH

A narrative is a coherent story with an identifiable beginning, middle and end that provides information about unanswered questions or unresolved conflict and provides a resolution. Applications of narrative to promote changes in health-related behaviours largely take the form of storytelling to convey informa-tion to other people. The individual or group summarises what has happened in the story, why it happened and what has been learned from this experience. This information is used to identify the causes of poor health and then to identify a means of addressing the issue. Digital storytelling is a modern format of the nar-rative approach that uses 3- to 5-minute visual narratives that synthesise images, video and audio recordings to create accounts of personal experience. Storytelling is especially effective when communicating with populations that have a strong oral tradition, a high level of illiteracy or both (Hinyard and Kreuter 2006). The narrative approach is based on a model developed by Paulo Freire (Freire 2005) in which the goal is to listen to the themes used in the story and to then create a dialogue. Everyone can participate in constructing a shared reality through the story which can lead to a transformation of ideas into actions (Gubrium 2009). Storytelling has been used to help survivors to discuss the reasons for refusing treatment and how they have coped with the stigma they have experienced. Working with survivors is discussed in Chapter 10.

Three traditional storytelling techniques that have been successfully used with communities are unserialised posters, three pile sorting cards and story with a gap.

## Unserialised posters

Unserialised posters are prepared in advance as pictures, for example, cuttings from magazines, photographs or hand-drawn diagrams. The pictures show a variety of situations relevant to the community such as an improved water supply about which the group members are asked to select four of the unserialised posters and to then develop a story by using the images. The group is asked to give names to the people and places in the pictures and to give the story a beginning, a middle and an end. The group is asked to present the story to other participants who are encouraged to ask questions. In particular, the facilitator should ask the following questions: Are these stories about events in your community? What issues have been raised that could be considered to be needs in your community? How could these be resolved? The facilitator keeps a record of the needs that have been identified during the presentation of the story. These points are then used to generate a discussion with the group on what it has learned and what needs it feels could be addressed by the community. The facilitator can help the community by developing a strategy to then address its concerns through identifying realistic actions and resources (Wood et al. 1998).

## Three-pile sorting cards

Three-pile sorting cards is a technique that can be used to develop a story about the causes of poor health as well as other problems in the community. A set of 15 cards, each with a picture that can be interpreted as either good, bad or in-between, from a health (or any other) perspective, are distributed among the participants. Some examples in regard to the prevention of the Zika virus are provided in the table below.

| Good | Bad | In-between |
| --- | --- | --- |
| Protective clothing | Mosquitos | Wearing shorts |
| Bed net | Mosquito biting | Drinking at night in bar |
| Insect repellent | Unprotected sex | Watching a pregnant mother |
| Condom | Holes in mosquito net | |

The task of the participants is to sort the 15 cards into each of the three categories (good, bad or in-between), reconsider their choices and then share their conclusions with the facilitator and with other group members. The participants are asked to select one or more cards from the bad category and create a list of actions to resolve the problems by using another selection of cards from the good category. The participants have to decide the reasons for the bad situation, who is responsible and how to address the issue: when, who and what is needed to address the issue. The participants can also identify potential partners to help them to address the issue such as a government agency, friends and family (Srinivasan 1993).

## The story with a gap

The story with a gap is an established approach that can be used to stimulate discussion about the needs of a community in a participatory way. Each group is given two large pictures. One picture shows the before situation of a community problem or need, for example, people living in a community with many mosquitoes. The second picture shows the after situation, for example, a healthy community with no mosquitoes or mosquito breeding places. The group is asked to develop a story which explains how this improvement has occurred. The stories that they develop will 'fill the gap' between the two pictures. The group members are asked to recount their story and the content is discussed to identify possible pathways to find solutions with the facilitator and with other group members (Srinivasan 1993).

# 4

# The risk communication approach

---

| KEY POINTS |
| --- |

- Risk communication can improve individual and collective prepared-ness, control and action to address disease outbreaks and health emergencies.
- Enabling people can be achieved by being a good communicator, a good listener and helping others to become more critically aware of their situation.
- A combination of different communication channels, as a part of the same campaign, can be a more effective approach to reinforce the key messages.
- Fear-based interventions are most effective when they are combined with a supportive environment that offers easy solutions to rectify risky behaviours.
- Volunteerism is possible at all levels so long as people are prepared to work together differently and to trust one another.

The importance of risk communication was highlighted during the release of anthrax in the United States in September 2001, the outbreak of severe acute respiratory syndrome (SARS) in Asia in 2003 and the H1N1 influenza pandemic in 2009. Public health emergencies have shown that a lack of planning, communication and community engagement can make an event potentially more dangerous (PREVENT 2011). Risk communication has traditionally been used to reduce public anxiety in regard to health threats or to manage people's awareness of the risks. A short coming has been that the public has not been fully involved from the start of the response through to its completion (Brennan and Gutierrez 2011). Not involving the public in a response runs the real risk of creating distrust, non-compliance and resistance.

> **BOX 4.1: The Tuskegee study**
>
> The Tuskegee study was conducted by the US public health service between 1932 and 1972 and involved 500 black sharecroppers and other men with untreated syphilis to document the course of the disease. The men were not told that they had syphilis and did not receive any counselling or treatment for the disease, even though since 1943 penicillin had been an effective drug. The study was brought to a halt under pressure from concerned researchers, but after an expert panel meeting it was allowed to continue to allow autopsies to be carried out. Eventually, those concerned went to the press and a media scandal ensued which brought the study to an end. The legacy has been that black and minority people have a mistrust of the medical profession which can act as a serious barrier to ongoing clinical projects (Cwikel 2006).

Best practice for risk communication should involve an interactive exchange of information among individuals, families and communities about the nature of a risk, to address concerns to messages or to legal and institutional arrangements (Committee on Risk Perception and Communication 1989). It is therefore a two-way process in which organisations communicate with the public, not at them, and engages with them to build constructive partnerships (Health Protection Network 2008).

> Risk communication can improve individual and collective preparedness, control and action to address disease outbreaks and health emergencies.

The ability to establish effective risk communication strategies will depend on whether the health promoter is perceived to be trustworthy. Trust and credibility, which are demonstrated through empathy and caring, competence and expertise, are essential elements of the risk communication approach (Reynolds and Crouse-Quinn 2008). Effective risk communication provides the public with information that enables them to make informed choices about how best to protect their health and to collaborate with agencies in identifying solutions to their problems (Covello and Allen 1998); therefore, trust is an essential ingredient.

## THE ROLE OF RISK COMMUNICATION

The role of risk communication is to address potential disease outbreaks and health emergencies by informing the individual and by engaging with and building community capacities towards greater resilience, empowerment and sustainability. Within a health promotion approach, there are two main types of actions that are used in risk communication: health education and social mobilisation.

# Health education

Health education is designed to target the individual to develop skills and to disseminate health-related knowledge. Health education provides the latest technical information to motivate people to change their unhealthy behaviours. It has traditionally relied on mass media campaigns because the frequency and design of communication activities have often been restricted by the poor availability of resources. Health education can also combine different communication channels as a part of the same campaign to reinforce the same key messages on a regular basis, for example, weekly radio broadcasts, the distribution of leaflets and house-to-house education. An 'opportunistic channel' can be included, such as a community event: an event that is used when the opportunity arises, usually when people congregate in a public place, for example, at clinics or in markets. A combination of channels can strengthen the approach; for example, didactic methods can be made more participatory when used with teaching aids such as flip charts. It is important that the stakeholders are clearly identified, the message content is specific and the materials are well presented and interesting (Laverack 2009).

The guiding principle of health education is to facilitate people to make informed choices about their behaviours. An informed choice is one that is based on relevant knowledge about a health behaviour and the perceived risk associated with a wrong choice, consistent with the decision maker's values and behaviour (Dormandy et al. 2002). The person volunteers to change his or her behaviour by identifying needs and then by taking actions to resolve them, such as improving the ability to perform a particular skill, for example, using personal protective

## BOX 4.2: Using communication for development to address Ebola in Guinea

Communities that were once considered off-limits to Ebola response teams in Guinea, West Africa, undertook their own outreach to help eradicate the disease. Getting communities to adopt safe behaviours, such as reporting sick people and allowing specialized teams to conduct burials, were critical. Outreach campaigns were conducted employing social mobilisers deployed across the country; radio stations broadcasting prevention messages; and traditional healers, religious leaders and women's organizations to spread messages. Although there was concern that some communities may have been hiding sick people or conducting unsafe burials, social mobilisers were able to engage, face to face, with health workers seeking to track down sick people or anyone who had been in contact with an infected person. One team identified a woman with suspected Ebola and were then able to convince her and her family to allow an ambulance to take her to a treatment centre, reducing the risk of cross-infection to the community (UNICEF 2015).

equipment to prevent the transmission of a disease. Different forms of communication such as the mass media, face-to-face education, social media and print materials can assist with the transfer of information and skills when working with both literate and non-literate populations. Visual images, for example, can be used to generate a two-way discussion between the health promoter and their clients and is especially useful in a teaching environment such as with school children.

> A combination of different communication channels, as a part of the same campaign, can be a more effective approach to reinforce the key messages.

## Social mobilisation

The purpose of social mobilization is to increase community action towards addressing a disease outbreak and health emergency. The outcome of social mobilisation is that individuals and communities are helped to gain greater control over decision-making and better access to resources in regard to health risks. Informed and autonomous choice is core to social mobilisation because it is the individual, group or community that is active in changing the circumstances. Autonomy refers to the capacity to be self-governing and making the decisions that will influence one's life and health. It is linked to what it is to be a person, to be able to choose freely and to be able to formulate how one wants to live one's life. It is also related to having the freedom and opportunities in our lives to be able to make the right choices for ourselves (Kant et al. 1997).

The actions of health education and social mobilisation must be delivered within a supportive environment, for example, with easy access to vaccination services. The actions should ideally have supportive legislation, for example, mandatory regulations for the vaccination of travellers. The actions must be underpinned by strong social support, such as positive normative values, and endorsed by faith and community leaders. Although these determinants are often outside of the control of health promoters, their achievement can be enhanced by supporting civil society action to influence the political context. The box below provides a case study of a risk communication approach in Egypt that used both health education and social mobilisation with the support of the national government.

## BOX 4.3: Preventing avian influenza in Egypt

In Egypt an intervention to prevent avian influenza (H5N1) identified several key success factors including multi-sectoral action and a multi-level implementation plan involving partners at the national, community and household levels. The intervention had a flexible approach that allowed for innovation as the disease outbreak changed. The health education strategy was delivered by the Ministry of Health to raise awareness and to avoid public concerns about the avian influenza outbreak. The key message themes included personal hygiene, the safe preparation of poultry, disease transmission and the proper care of caged birds. These messages were transmitted through the mass media and variety of printed materials such as leaflets and via face-to-face communication by health professionals including pharmacists. The intervention achieved a coverage of 85% of households in the first phase; however, further analysis showed that although most people accepted that there was a threat from avian influenza, they did not believe that it would affect their households. The Ministry of Health then decided that a new social mobilisation approach was required in the second phase to increase the perception of risk and to motivate people to address the threat at the household level. This began with voluntary community mapping exercises, door-to-door messaging and peer education interventions. The combination of the use of mass media and community-based activities helped to increase safer caging practices and personal protective behaviours. The analysis showed that those villages that participated in the community-based activities had a greater rate of behaviour change than those that did not and that had only relied on the mass media campaign (Bertrand et al. 2011).

## RISK FACTORS

Risk factors refer to the social, economic and biological status; behaviours; and environments which are associated with or cause increased susceptibility to a specific disease, ill health or injury. Once risk factors have been identified, they can become the entry point or focus for health promotion strategies and actions (WHO 1998).

Understanding the risks to health is key to preventing disease outbreaks. However, a particular disease is often caused by more than one risk factor, which means that multiple interventions are needed; for example, *Mycobacterium tuberculosis* is the direct cause of tuberculosis, but overcrowded housing and poor nutrition also increase the risk of infection, which presents multiple paths for preventing the disease. In turn, most risk factors are associated with more than one disease and targeting those factors can reduce multiple causes of disease. For example, reducing tobacco smoking will result in fewer deaths and less disease from lung cancer and other chronic respiratory diseases (WHO 2009a).

Psychosocial risk factors describe individual cognitive or emotional states such as self-esteem which are often reactions to risk conditions and which also influence our desire and ability to create social networks. The stress, for example, created by the loss of a family member can become physical pathology. People living in high-risk conditions such as a disease outbreak experience distress and internalise the unfairness of the situation. This internalisation adds to their distress with measurable effects on their bodies, or physiological risk factors. People caught in the cycle of risk conditions and risk factors

## BOX 4.4: Risk factors and disease outbreaks

In 1847, the Prussian province of Silesia was ravaged by a typhoid epidemic. Because the crisis threatened the population of coal miners in the area, and thus the economy, the Prussian government hired the young pathologist Rudolf Virchow to investigate the problem. He spent 3 weeks living with the miners and their families. One of the first points he made in his report was that typhoid was only one of several diseases afflicting the coal miners, with dysentery, measles and tuberculosis being other diseases. Virchow referred to these diseases as 'artificial' to emphasise that although they had their origin with a particular and 'naturally' occurring bacterium, their epidemic rates in Silesia were determined by poor housing, working conditions, diet and lack of sanitation among the coal miners. To facilitate people realising their own needs, he proposed a joint committee involving both lay people and professionals. This group would monitor the spread of typhoid and other diseases while organizing agricultural food cooperatives to ensure the people had sufficient food to eat. To Virchow, all disease has two causes: one pathological and the other political. Virchow's story tells us that diseases are physiological events that arise within, and derive their meaning or significance from, particular social and political contexts. It foreshadows the important role played by educated, empowered and organized groups of citizens in creating healthy social change. Infectious diseases declined dramatically in industrialised countries at the end of the last century, a transition in large part resulting from social and political changes such as improved sanitation, improved working and living conditions, improved nutrition and family planning. These changes did not come easily because employers opposed sanitary reforms and quarantines on imported goods because they reduced profits (Taylor and Rieger 1985).

usually experience less social support and greater isolation and are less likely to be active in groups concerned with improving their circumstances. This then reinforces their sense of isolation and self-blame, reinforcing the experience of disease outbreak. Health professionals may begin their work with an individual or group around a physiological, behavioural or psychosocial risk factor. Once risk factors have been identified, these can become the focus for a risk communication intervention. But health professionals must also identify the risk conditions, otherwise they will only treat the symptoms and not prevent the cause of the health problem. The task is to locate these diseases and behavioural risks in their psychosocial and socioenvironmental contexts, for example, powerlessness, poverty and isolation, and to recognize these contexts as independent health risks in their own right.

# STRENGTHENING RISK COMMUNICATION

Risk communication can best be strengthened at the national level through a strategic framework that includes the following areas:

1. The development of staff skills, in particular, for community mobilisation to identify needs, build capacity and gain more control over preparedness to deal with risks
2. The development of tools and methodologies for risk communication
3. Training and competence for organisational development

The way forward is to strengthen a national risk communication framework to better respond to public needs in regard to disease outbreaks and, in particular, to have clear roles and responsibilities for involving the community (World Health Organization 2016f).

# INVOLVING THE COMMUNITY

The risk communication approach must go beyond simply providing information. A two-way dialogue between the response agency and the public must be established to encourage community participation in the process of planning and decision-making. This can be achieved in three phases: (1) preparation, (2) response and control and (3) recovery.

## Preparation phase

It is important to assess, coordinate, plan and listen to others because this provides the opportunity for them to help to control a potential disease outbreak.

---

**BOX 4.5: Risk communication and foot and mouth disease**

New Zealand's Ministry of Agriculture and Forestry (MAF) provided a response to a letter claiming that activists had released the foot and mouth disease virus in 2005 into the environment. The financial impact would have been devastating for New Zealand and its farming community. Animals were tested and the feasibility of infecting the cattle in the precise manner described in the threatening letter was subjected to rigorous scientific debate. The MAF engaged with the farming community in New Zealand and took steps together by using counter tactics to declare the event a hoax within a week. The MAF's patient and thorough response allowed the agency to maintain the confidence of New Zealand's citizens and the international marketplace. New Zealand's farmers saw no lasting impact of the event on consumption and exportation of their product (CDC 2012).

Building an effective dialogue with the public is an important aspect of the preparation phase including their participation to share experiences and to recruit their voluntary services. Participation is essential because it allows people to become involved in activities which influence their lives and health. This can be enhanced by actively recruiting people to volunteer to assist in a disease outbreak. The outside agency has opportunities to involve the community including meetings or forums to discuss issues and to disseminate information. The meeting or forum would typically begin with a brief introduction to the purpose and a focus on a particular risk. The meeting can be used to plan for actions and identify resources and potential partners and for people to openly express their views and concerns.

Engagement is a collaborative process, often between a risk communication agency and the community, involving people in identifying needs and solutions to risks that affect their lives. The success of a risk communication campaign depends on the commitment and involvement of the public. People are much more likely to be committed if they have a sense of ownership in regard to the solutions being used to address an outbreak and if these solutions also meet their own needs. Community stories, for example, can be used to identify important risk communication needs and can be initiated through group discussion and the voicing of experiences. Community stories involve others to identify important needs and to help build a mutual understanding of the outcomes (Wood et al. 1998). Various techniques can be used to stimulate the process of developing a story including using photographs or encouraging the participants to draw a picture. People describe their experiences by using these techniques, and this in turn provides more meaning and context. This is discussed in Chapter 3.

> Enabling people can be achieved by being a good communicator, a good listener and helping others to become more critically aware of their situation.

Risk communication that does not address public needs and that does not involve communities runs the real risk of not achieving its purpose. The identification of needs, solutions and actions must be carried out in close collaboration with the community. To reach conclusions about the risks, the public can access information from a variety of sources including the mass media, the internet, friends and family (Allmark and Tod 2006). Health promoters have traditionally used simple, one-way messaging that may exaggerate the risks of a particular behaviour or the benefits of changing that behaviour. An over-reliance on these approaches has led to mistrust in the public, people feel that risk does not apply to them and they can reject the advice (Hunt and Emslie 2001). Conflicting sources of information can also make people feel more at risk; for example, in the UK public concerns were raised about the measles, mumps and rubella vaccine. The health authorities saw this as an effective option with few side effects. However, after media reports of conflicting scientific evidence the public became increasingly concerned that the vaccine could lead to bowel cancer and autism.

These concerns were confounded by the past distrust between the authorities and the public over the handling of the outbreak of bovine spongiform encephalopathy (mad cow disease) and conflicting evidence on the benefits of screening (Smith 2002).

## Response and control phase

It is important to address the outbreak using a strategic plan to build local capacity and to work with others in partnership to both disseminate key messages and to promote social mobilisation. Community capacity building is the increase in community groups' abilities to define, assess, analyse and act on health (or any other) concerns of importance to their members. More generally, it is viewed as a process that increases the assets and attributes that a community is able to draw upon (Goodman et al. 1998). Community capacity building is not specific to a particular locality, or to the individuals or groups within it, but to the interactions between both. Community capacity building is achieved through systematically building knowledge, skills and competencies at an individual and collective levels and can be unpacked into the organisational areas of influence that significantly contribute to its development.

## Recovery phase

It is important to share the lessons learnt and to identify actions to enable people to have the skills and capacity to address future outbreaks. A goal of the risk communication approach is to improve collective and individual decision-making (Covello and Allen 1998). People work to increase their control over decisions that determine the effects of a health risk in their lives. Empowerment embodies the notion that an increase in control must come from within an individual, group or community and cannot be given to them. This is achieved through the facilitation of capacity building: an increase in knowledge, skills and competencies. The role of the health promoter, at the request of the community, is to help build capacity and provide resources, information and skills training to individuals, groups and communities. This can be achieved in small groups or community organisations that are able to act collectively such as by conducting a rapid needs assessment. Later, the community can develop stronger networks towards preparedness and action for an outbreak response.

## FEAR-BASED INTERVENTIONS

A fear-based intervention uses the threat of harmful consequences to the target audience for starting or continuing a particular high-risk behaviour (Corcoran 2013). Fear-based interventions are implemented as a component of communication approaches, for example, using graphic images to dissuade people from using unsafe practices (Corcoran 2013). Fear-based interventions use persuasion based on aspects of disgust and rational reasoning of perceived risk to change people's beliefs and behaviours. Persuasion is a process aimed at changing individual or group attitudes, beliefs or behaviours by using methods of communication to convey information, feelings or reasoning (Seiter and Gass 2010).

In practice, it cannot be assumed that using fear-based tactics such as graphic images or messages will automatically lead to a positive change in behaviour. One study, for example, showed that negative campaigns using an element of fear in a social marketing strategy, designed to increase compliance, were more likely to invoke inaction rather than an active response such as volunteering to comply (Brennan and Binney 2010). In another study involving 840 young adults, the use of fear-based campaigns changed participants' beliefs about distractions caused by four unsafe behaviours. After viewing two fear-based interventions, participants reported increased intentions of actually engaging in the behaviours, especially the males, and aroused only low-to-moderate levels of fear. The study concluded that the fear-based intervention was not effective in changing attitude or practices in young adults in regard to safer behaviours (Lennon et al. 2010). A meta-analysis of fear-based HIV prevention interventions found that the strategy did not work to increase the rate of condom use and that such approaches may actually be associated with decreases in condom use. Appealing to people's fears, for example, in regard to HIV prevention may work better on people who are well equipped to change their behaviour, for example, those that already have a high self-efficacy and are well resourced, psychologically and socially, to process the messages and to change their behaviour. Those people who are less equipped to adopt the recommended behaviour may be made to feel worse, and the fear-based intervention can then lead to behaviours that increase their risk (Albarracin et al. 2005).

Strategies designed to invoke fear, guilt and shame can confuse the recipients or create feelings of powerlessness and inaction. Fear-based interventions can have a negative effect where the audience reaction is the opposite to the intended effect of the message. Messaging must therefore be rigorously tested with the target audiences to ensure it produces the intended changes in awareness, attitude, and behavioural intention. Health promoters should also ensure that interventions are backed up with a supportive environment to enable people to act upon the messages, including those who have strong defensive reactions and those who feel that the intervention is irrelevant to their own lives (Thomas et al. 2014).

> Fear-based interventions are most effective when they are combined with a supportive environment that offers easy solutions to rectify risky behaviours.

## WORKING WITH VOLUNTEERS AND LAY HEALTH WORKERS

Volunteering can be defined as an activity that involves spending time doing something for free that aims to benefit others including relatives (Volunteering England 2012). Volunteerism is an important aspect of working with communities and is an activity that can produce feelings of self-respect, skills development and socialization. An important distinction is between the participation of individual volunteers and the voluntary and community sector which provides an infrastructure for citizen involvement across the third sector. The third sector is a term used to cover all not-for-profit organisations: voluntary, community charities; and social non-government associations. There is a wide array of terms that can be used to describe volunteer roles including community health advocates and educators, link workers, peer coaches and counsellors, community champions and popular opinion leaders.

In particular, lay health workers have been an effective means to engage communities in disease outbreaks by actively involving them in organizing, peer education, as opinion leaders and to act as a link between communities and health services (South et al. 2013). Lay health workers are members of the communities where they work, selected by the communities, answerable to the communities for their activities, supported by the health system but not necessarily part of its organization (World Health Organization 2007).

> Volunteerism is possible at all levels so long as people are prepared to work together differently and to trust one another.

Volunteers are sometimes trained in the areas they work, such as education and counselling, whereas others can serve on a casual basis, such as in outreach activities, culturally sensitive care, home visiting and helping with transportation.

Volunteering often plays a pivotal role in community interventions because they can provide a valuable network of local contacts and social support (Winfield 2013). Many community-based organisations depend on the hard-working efforts of volunteers who, behind the scenes, strive tirelessly doing day-to-day activities. These volunteers receive no or low pay, and one of the most critical problems for volunteerism is the high rate of attrition that can

## BOX 4.6: Volunteerism in Sierra Leone

Small teams of volunteer social mobilisers were used to enter communities in Sierra Leone that were under a 21-day quarantine after recording an Ebola death. These volunteer 'hotspot busters' were deployed rapidly to communities considered high risk for Ebola transmission and were trained to intensify social mobilisation activities and increase the engagement of communities. They conducted one-on-one sensitisation sessions, house-to-house visits and public awareness-raising activities. They encouraged community members to call the 117 Ebola hotline to report sick people who were then referred to a healthcare facility. They worked with youth, women and volunteer networks to reach as many households as possible (UNICEF 2015a).

lead to a lack of continuity in the relationship between the programme and the community. This attrition increases costs and time in selecting and training new volunteers. Good leadership, communication and self-reflection are therefore key aspects in helping to maintain voluntary action (Frusciante 2007).

An international review of lay health workers found that successful projects had multiple incentives to provide better job satisfaction. Incentives did not have to be monetary but were often in-kind such as clothing or an appreciation of their role through greater professional support. The review concluded that the sustainability of voluntary inputs depended on several key factors including:

- Volunteers should maintain a relationship with the community but remain accountable to them for their activities.
- The programme should plan for a high turnover of volunteers, for example, by having shorter but more regular training.
- Volunteers should continue to be made to feel valued by the health system and to collaborate with other health professionals, for example, in outreach activities.
- The spirit of volunteerism should be maintained for as long as possible, and when incentives are introduced they should be multiple and matched to duties and responsibilities.
- Regular monitoring of duties and providing feedback to the volunteers (Bhattacharya et al. 2001).

However, the high attrition rates, the need for regular training, multiple incentives and the monitoring of duties mean that volunteerism is not always a cost-effective option for health promotion interventions in disease outbreaks.

# 5

# Engaging with communities

---

## KEY POINTS

- A systematic and structured approach to community engagement is essential to build trust and to promote participation.
- A needs assessment is a logical starting point in the design of any health promotion programme to build long-term working relationships.
- Partnerships are a pivotal point at which people increase their control over a range of issues that influence their health.
- Empowerment can be achieved through systematically building knowledge, skills and competencies to give people more control at a local level.
- Respect for the local culture and recognition of community autonomy to plan and implement their own actions are crucial to the success of a response.

## WHAT IS 'COMMUNITY'?

As a working 'rule of thumb' a community will occupy a spatial dimension, such as a village or a virtual space or place, and a non-spatial dimension that involves relationships between people. Within the geographic dimensions of a community, multiple sub-communities often exist and individuals may belong to several of these 'interest groups' at the same time. Interest groups exist as a legitimate means by which individuals are organised around a variety of social activities, for example, funerals, or to address a shared concern, for example, the lack of healthcare services (Zakus and Lysack 1998). However, the diversity of interests within a community can sometimes create problems, and health promoters must try to avoid the establishment of a dominant minority that can dictate issues based only on their concerns and not those of the broader community.

> A systematic and structured approach to community engagement is essential to build trust and to promote participation.

Civil society goes beyond the concept of a 'community' to include people in both their social and professional contexts and stresses the need for a developed level of public and political participation, both of which are central to health promotion. Civil society works through people who create groups, organisations, communities and movements to address shared needs. Civil societies are populated by organisations such as registered charities, non-government organisations, women's organisations, faith-based organisations, trade unions, self-help groups, social movements and activist and advocacy groups (Laverack 2014).

## WORKING IN DIFFERENT SETTINGS

A setting is a place or social context in which people engage in daily activities and in which environmental, organisational and personal factors interact to affect health and well-being (World Health Organization 1998). Settings can normally be identified as having physical boundaries, a range of people with defined roles and an organisational structure. Settings provide a convenient means for health promotion activities during a disease outbreak and include schools, workplaces, communities and hospitals. Settings can be used to promote health by reaching people who occupy them, raising awareness, developing skills, gaining better access to services, changing the physical environment or strengthening organisational structures (Naidoo and Wills 2009). In a school setting, for example, health promoters are able to engage health and education officials, teachers, students, parents and health providers in response efforts. The setting can also provide a link between the school and the local community to help understand their roles in the disease outbreak (World Health Organization 1997a).

### Working in urban neighbourhoods

Working in urban neighbourhoods requires a specific strategy of engagement, starting with the city authorities and a consideration of existing by-laws. This may involve discussing how some of the by-laws will be applied during an outbreak such as the positioning of latrines, treatment centres and distribution points. Communal emergency toilets and other facilities can also be constructed to improve sanitation with the support of the local administrative authorities. Working in urban neighbourhoods to address disease outbreaks is a unique challenge and is a very different setting to a rural community. The UNMEER/UN-Habitat intervention in Montserrado, Monrovia, for example, used approaches that first engaged with local officials within administrative boundaries in urban areas to address the Ebola outbreak in Liberia (Laverack and Manoncourt 2015). The Ebola virus receded from the rural areas into the urban areas during the final phases of the outbreak. In densely populated areas, such as refugee camps and urban slums, an outbreak can spread quickly because of the high population density, facilitating person-to-person transmission (Lamond and Kinjanyui 2012). However, a standard operational procedure for community engagement in urban neighbourhoods, although used in some localised settings, was not extensively shared across the three affected countries.

Poor economic environments and unstable living conditions, insufficient water supply, inadequate sanitation and hygiene and high population density create favourable factors for the spread of disease among the most vulnerable. Slum areas often have fragile health and education services and social mobilisation can be impeded due to the resistance of the residents, who may be illegally occupying their living spaces. Households cannot be quarantined individually because of a lack of space, so responders try to place whole neighbourhoods under quarantine. This can create resistance about issues such as latrines being shared between quarantined and non-quarantined households. The fragile situation in densely populated urban neighbourhoods can be further exasperated by the forceful tactics used by authorities; for example, the military was used in West Point, Liberia, to impose a quarantine in August 2014. This quickly led to riots and deaths, and the quarantine had to be stopped by the authorities (ACAPS 2015).

## THE COMMUNITY ENGAGEMENT FRAMEWORK

Before starting the process of community engagement, it is useful for the health promoter to consider the following questions to better understand the context and purpose of the activity.

### What is the purpose of the community engagement?

Community engagement is usually initiated and led by an outside agency which controls the situation, for example, through identifying the key issues to be addressed. Community engagement can be wrongly used to coerce the community into participating in the activities of the outbreak response without identifying local needs or building their capacity towards local action. The key issue is whether the outside agents want to help to empower the community or to simply have them participate in the programme that they are employed to deliver.

### Is there a working definition of community engagement?

Westernised concepts such as community engagement can have different interpretations in other cultural contexts. How relevant are these terms to the lives and work of other stakeholders, particularly to communities? It is better to use terms that have been identified by the stakeholders themselves because lay interpretations can be used as an alternative to technical terminology. The purpose is to provide all stakeholders with a more mutual understanding of the programme in which they are involved and towards which they are expected to contribute. The identification of a working definition of the key terms used in the programme can be developed during the design phase by using qualitative techniques (see Chapter 2) and carried out involving the members of the community, with the assistance of the health promoter.

**Is it necessary to work with a cross-cultural team?**

The unfamiliarity with a specific cultural context can make it more difficult for health promoters to understand the reality of the situation, and this can influence the delivery of the response. A team comprising both foreign personnel and facilitators from the host country or community can provide the most suitable approach in a cross-cultural context. When it is not possible to work in a team, or if a local person is not available, then adequate training about the cultural context should be provided to everyone (Russon 1995). It is also important for the outside agent to have a prior understanding of the complex balance of relationships that occur between programme stakeholders in a cross-cultural context. Activities that may seem to have little relevance, such as the seating arrangements in a meeting, may have profound implications for some members of the community. This understanding can be improved through cross-cultural awareness training, anthropological information and better communication (Cass et al. 2002).

> Invest in trusted local organisations and networks to facilitate community engagement and to reach a wide audience through face-to-face communication to transfer messages.

The community engagement framework is a systematic procedure of communication, engagement and feedback that can be used in a disease outbreak. The community engagement framework uses a systematic approach as follows: stakeholder connection, communication, needs assessment, informing the wider community, strengthening community capacity, building partnerships and follow-up (Figure 5.1).

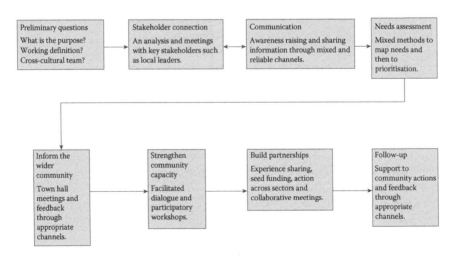

Figure 5.1 The community engagement framework.

## Stakeholder connection

There is a relationship between the health promoter and the range of people with whom they work, including those people who are directly affected by the response and people who may act to inhibit the response or may be super-spreaders of the disease. Different terms are used to describe these people including the primary stakeholders, the target audience and the community. These are the partners at whom the services, information and resources are targeted and include women, adolescents and men, and different socioeconomic and cultural groups. These people occupy different settings, for example, social groups, schools and hospitals. Other partners act as an intermediary in the delivery of the programme, for example, health promotion agencies and the health promoters that they employ (Laverack 2009). The key partners are identified during the planning phase and according to the requirements of the programme may be further categorised by age, gender, marital status, ethnicity and socioeconomic background. The programme may also specifically target marginalised groups that can become excluded from preventive, treatment and rehabilitation services.

## Communication

Health communication is a key strategy to inform the public, maintain their involvement in the programme and protect and improve their health status. Health communication uses many approaches including edutainment, health journalism, interpersonal communication, advocacy, risk communication, social marketing and traditional and culture-specific activities such as storytelling, puppet shows and songs.

Successful communication campaigns have achieved improvements in the level of awareness and have changed specific behaviours by using social marketing, peer education and the social media, as discussed in Chapter 3. However, the evidence is mixed seemingly working in some contexts, but not in others, and communication campaigns must use a comprehensive approach by including a range of techniques that are culturally appropriate and that reinforce the key health messages.

## Needs assessment

Needs assessment is used to identify the needs reported by an individual, group or community and the resources and outcomes that are required to address them (Gilmore 2011). A needs assessment should be the starting point of every programme and include an identification of assets and the development of activities based on people's capabilities, knowledge and skills. Mapping is an important stage in needs assessment and includes engaging with an 'audience', the identification, ranking and prioritization of their concerns. It helps to create an inventory of the strengths and the social interconnections of people and how these can be accessed. This is important because the opportunities for health promotion are to a large extent dependent on social, financial, physical and environmental assets at a local level (Jirojwong and Liamputtong 2009). The response also has needs that it may wish to address, typically based on health data. Sometimes, these are similar to those of the community and can be reconciled in the design of the programme otherwise a compromise has to be found through the implementation of the response.

> A needs assessment is a logical starting point in the design of any health promotion programme to build long-term working relationships.

Needs assessment involves quantitative as well as qualitative methods to determine priorities, what should be done, what can be done and what can be afforded. However, too rigid an approach runs the risk of becoming too controlling, whereas too flexible an approach runs the risk of delay or not having a direction with which to move forward (Wright 2001). In practice, who will participate in the needs assessment is essentially decided through the representation of a few partners on behalf of the majority, for example, the elected representatives of a community. This is because it is not usually possible for everyone to participate in the needs assessment even when using participatory methods. The diversity of some communities can create problems with regard to the intentional exclusion of specific groups, including the exclusion of women. The participation can then become empty and frustrating for those whose involvement is passive and can have a negative effect on the success of an outbreak response. Participation can also allow those in authority, for example, the programme management, to claim that all sides were considered, whereas only a few benefit. The approach used must therefore include the felt needs of all people affected by the outbreak.

## Informing the wider community

It is important to inform the wider community about the progress and problems faced by the response. Communities play an important role in disease outbreaks through, for example, self-quarantines, contact tracing and complying with advice on hygiene and vector control. It is therefore crucial that they are involved in the dissemination of information and in regular updates on the progress of the outbreak response. This can be achieved through the sharing of relevant information through regular forums and the use of appropriate communication channels, including social media and radio broadcasts.

> ### BOX 5.1: Informing the wider community during a foot and mouth outbreak
>
> During the 2001 foot and mouth emergency in the UK, there was considerable concern over the health issues surrounding the disposal of animal carcasses. Three regional teams of government officials were headed by the Regional Directors of Public Health. Public meetings in the most affected areas were held to consult with local communities

to reassure people about the local health risks. The local Public Health Director, selected for respect and trust, led the team meetings. Before the public meeting, informal contact with local opinion leaders was made to ensure that the real issues were being tackled. Teams were provided with a briefing, which was regularly updated, and included a response to public questions and rumours. A 'Mobile Communication Unit' toured the affected areas and delivered basic advice as well as information leaflets, which were also distributed to the public through the public meetings and at shopping centres (Cabinet office 2011).

## Strengthen community capacity

Capacity building is the process by which the end result of increasing sustainability can be achieved through strengthening the knowledge, skills and competencies of the community. Community capacity building increases people's abilities to define, assess, analyse and act on health (or any other) concerns of importance to themselves (Labonte and Laverack 2001). Recently, this concept has been 'unpacked' into nine 'capacity domains' that represent those aspects that allow people to better organise and mobilise themselves towards gaining greater control over their lives. Capacities in each of the domains can be indicative of a robust and capable community, one that has strong organisational and social abilities. The nine capacity domains are as follows: improve stakeholder participation, develop local leadership, build organisational structures, increase problem assessment capacities, enhance stakeholder ability to 'ask why', improve resource mobilisation, strengthen links to other organisations and people, create an equitable relationship with outside agents, and increase stakeholder control over programme management. One participatory approach to build community capacity uses the nine domains to enable people to better organise themselves, to strategically plan for actions to resolve their concerns and to evaluate the outcomes, as follows:

- A period of observation and discussion is important to first adapt the approach to the social and cultural requirements of the participants. For example, the use of a working definition of community capacity building can provide all participants with a more mutual understanding of the concept in which they are involved and towards which they are expected to contribute.
- Measurement is in itself insufficient to build capacity, so this information must also be transformed into actions. This is achieved through strategic planning for positive changes in the nine domains to achieve improvements at an individual and a community level based on the following: identifying specific activities; sequencing activities into the correct order to make an improvement; setting a realistic time frame, including any targets; and assigning individual responsibilities to complete each activity within the programme time frame.
- The resources that are necessary and available to improve the present situation are assessed (Laverack 2007).

# Building partnerships

Partnerships demonstrate the ability of a community to develop relationships with different organisations to better collaborate and cooperate. They may involve an exchange of services, pursuit of a joint venture based on a shared goal or an advocacy initiative to change policy. The purpose of a partnership is to grow beyond local concerns and to take a stronger position on broader issues through networking and resource mobilisation. A key issue is that the members of the partnership are able to remain focused on the shared need that brings them together, and not on the individual needs in the partnership (Laverack 2004). The role of the health promoter is to help to develop partnerships in regard to a potential risk. Partnerships help to build the capacity of the community through an expanded membership and resource base. In turn, this provides communities with the ability to have greater collective influence, participation and resource mobilisation.

Key lessons learnt from using partnerships in health promotion do recur and can be summarised as follows:

- Many partnership forums are simply information exchanging networks which, although helpful in a limited way, are a questionable use of both government and community resources.
- The financial, logistical and time costs of effective partnerships can be large and engaging across sectors should be done with clarity of purpose.
- Ensuring that partners have overlapping interests in the disease outbreak is essential to establish some shared action.
- Resources do not always have to be financial and may involve an intimate knowledge of the causes and consequences of the disease outbreak. However, the willingness of members to pool resources, primarily finances, can be a motivating feature for new initiatives (Labonte and Laverack 2008).

> Partnerships are a pivotal point at which people increase their control over a range of issues that influences their health.

Fundamental to building multi-sectoral partnerships is the involvement of the key actors not only from within the health sector but also from other sectors that have an influence on the disease outbreak. Below is a case study of multi-sectoral action to address the control of avian flu in Turkey.

## BOX 5.2: Multi-sectoral action and avian flu

The Turkish experience of addressing avian flu demonstrates the need for proper planning and preparedness to be carried out at the international, national and local levels. Early national planning helped Turkey establish mechanisms for rapid problem-solving, multi-sectoral committees, surveillance and social mobilisation. The remote location of the avian flu outbreak in Turkey in January 2006, combined with exceptionally harsh weather, created the need for a decentralised response that can be summarised by the following:

1. Political leadership focusing on difficult issues.
2. A whole of government approach, as well as the private and voluntary sectors.
3. Mass media campaigns.
4. Key people made responsible and accountable at national and local levels.
5. Incentives and compensation schemes to reduce vulnerability.
6. Regular reviews of progress by all stakeholders.
7. Community involvement in support of the national action plan. In the outbreak, strengthening working relationships between the health and veterinary sectors was essential because the cause of the infection was linked directly to the interaction between poultry and humans. Attention to equity was also essential because most people in poor rural areas in Turkey keep poultry and created the epicentre of the outbreak. In Turkey the outbreak clarified the weakness in the ability of the national preparedness plan to cover remote and socially isolation communities (World Health Organization 2006).

## Follow-up

The follow-up step involves supporting and encouraging communities and sharing relevant information about available services and resources. Follow-up should use appropriate channels of communication and can include regular meetings with community and religious leaders and local community boards, household visits and text messaging. The purpose is to maintain contact with the community, inform them and ensure their continued support for ongoing activities in the outbreak response.

## COMMUNITY ENGAGEMENT AND CLINICAL TRIALS

The World Health Organization (WHO 2012a) defines a clinical trial as any research study that prospectively assigns human participants or groups of humans to one or more health-related interventions to evaluate the effects on health outcomes. Clinical trials are commonly classified into four phases. Each phase is treated separately, and the trial will normally proceed through all four phases over many years:

1. Clinical trials test a new biomedical intervention in a small group of people (e.g. 20–80) for the first time to evaluate safety (e.g. to determine a safe dosage range and to identify side effects).

2. Clinical trials study the biomedical or behavioural intervention in a larger group of people (several hundred) to determine efficacy and to further evaluate its safety.
3. Studies investigate the efficacy of the biomedical or behavioural intervention in large groups of human subjects (from several hundred to several thousand) by comparing the intervention to other standard or experimental interventions as well as monitoring adverse effects and collecting information that will allow the intervention to be used safely.
4. Studies are conducted after the intervention has been marketed. These studies are designed to monitor effectiveness of the approved intervention in the general population and to collect information about any adverse effects associated with widespread use.

Clinical trials can also randomly assign the intervention or vaccine to either of two groups:

1. The treatment group which uses the treatment or vaccine being assessed
2. The control group which uses an existing standard treatment, or a placebo, if no proven standard treatment exists

Although the treatments are different in the two groups, researchers will try to keep as many of the other conditions the same as possible. For example, both groups should have people of a similar age, with a similar proportion of men and women, who are in similar overall health.

The clinical trial will use a 'blinding' technique to ensure that no one in the study knows who has been assigned the intervention treatment, a standard treatment or the placebo to reduce the effects of bias when comparing the outcomes. The aim of the trial is to compare what happens in each group. The results have to be different enough between the two groups to prove that the difference has not just occurred by chance. If the individuals in the group being given the new intervention show a significant improvement, without any serious side effects, over the control group, then the researchers may end the clinical trial early and seek to change the nature of the clinical trial to afford more patients the opportunity to receive the new intervention.

## Engaging with the study community

The testing of vaccines in clinical trials requires an appropriate population group to participate in the study. A clinical trial that proceeds without established knowledge of the cultural nuances that affects their perceptions about health, infection and vaccinations could potentially create resistance to participate in the study. Rumours can also affect the uptake of vaccination. Polio eradication in northern Nigeria and Pakistan, for example, has been hindered by poor community trust. Communities want to engage in the agenda setting that governs the clinical trial, but the urgency often surrounding a vaccine development study can preclude correct community engagement.

## BOX 5.3: Community engagement in Ebola vaccine trials

The EBOVAC-Salone study is one of several vaccine trials set up in West Africa during and after the Ebola virus disease epidemic. The EBOVAC-Salone study aims to assess the safety and immunogenicity of the Ad26.ZEBOV/MVA-BN-Filo prime-boost regimen in a population affected by Ebola. The study, in the Kambia District in northern Sierra Leone, faced difficulties in identifying people to participate in the study and developed three complementary approaches for community liaison in supporting the establishment of the Ebola vaccine trial: a community engagement strategy, identification tools to ensure correct administration of the investigational vaccine and mobile technology to reinforce engagement and awareness (Enria et al. 2016).

### A COMMUNITY ENGAGEMENT STRATEGY

Local people were recruited and trained to be a part of the engagement teams interacting with the Kambia community. These community liaison officers worked closely with the local authorities and communities to build awareness and address potential rumours related to the vaccine study. Community engagement strategies included house-to-house visits and public meetings with key stakeholders supported by posters, leaflets and flip charts that were developed with artwork from local artists. The flip charts, for example, were used to explain the informed consent process to the volunteers for the study.

### IDENTIFICATION TOOLS TO ENSURE CORRECT ADMINISTRATION

Ensuring the right volunteer receives both a prime and boost of the investigational vaccine regimen at the right time required the implementation of an innovative state-of-the-art identification technology. Taking into consideration cultural acceptance, a dedicated team developed a solution based on validated fingerprinting and an iris scan technology that enables positive recognition of the study participants. Access to printer technology ensured that laminated vaccination cards could be made locally, and the whole technology package was portable and can operate independently for up to 8 hours.

### MOBILE TECHNOLOGY TO REINFORCE ENGAGEMENT AND AWARENESS

Community engagement requires the use of multiple communication tools that can facilitate wide-ranging procedures within the time available to conduct the study. To ensure volunteers remain engaged with the study and attend clinic visits, EBODAC created a mobile application to send customised messages to consenting volunteers that have a mobile phone. They received voice reminders in four local languages or in English about their clinic visit and about vaccine-related information ensuring they remained engaged in the study. The mobile technology platform also supported the vaccination team by providing a list of participants expected to attend a study visit.

This process ensures that the community members are consulted at the beginning of the study in an open, collaborative way. The basic principle is that before the clinical trial begins the design should be acceptable to the community hosting the study.

Healthcare providers are also a critical 'community' to engage with during a vaccine clinical trial. For example, the 'Ring' methodology in vaccine research studies uses a contact-tracing approach to first identify people known to have been in contact with a diagnosed index case and then offer them vaccination. Ideally, they should be engaged at an early stage to provide information and to gain their consent in the trial. Failure to actively engage healthcare providers in the study design may result in the slow recruitment of study participants due to misconceptions, stigma and fear. The recruitment of healthcare workers in one Ebola vaccine study, for example, did result in the coercion of initially dissenting workers to assist in the management of infected persons due to mistaken beliefs that the vaccine offered protection. The possibility of the study participants contracting Ebola infection, despite the use of an experimental vaccine, and the standard of care they would receive, needed to be clearly addressed and formalised as part of the ethics review and the process of engagement (Folayan et al. 2016).

## COMMUNITY EMPOWERMENT

Empowerment in the broadest sense is the process by which disadvantaged people work together to increase control over events that determine their lives (Werner 1988). As a process, community empowerment has been consistently viewed in the literature as a 5-point continuum comprised of the following elements: personal action, small groups, community organisations, partnerships, and social and political action. The continuum of community empowerment can help us to understand the potential that people have to progress from individual to collective action (Figure 5.2).

If a way forward is not possible the process can stop or move back to the preceding point on the continuum. The development of a community organisation is pivotal because it is the point at which small groups are able to make the transition to a broader organisational structure. However, it is through partnerships that people are able to gain a greater participant and resource base to influence other stakeholders in the disease outbreak. However, organisations can be quickly created in the response and may flourish for a time and then fade away

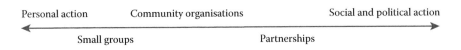

Figure 5.2 The continuum of community empowerment. (Laverack, 1999, p. 92).

for reasons as much to do with changes in the lack of political or financial support or a change in the nature of the health emergency. The role of health promoters is to work with the different levels on the continuum in ways that can help people to become more active in collective action. Community empowerment and community engagement overlap as forms of social mobilisation that involve people becoming better organised to address an issue. In a response context, capacity building is the means by which an outcome of empowerment can be achieved through systematically building knowledge, skills and competencies at a local level and by engaging with the different stakeholders to help to improve their lives.

> Empowerment can be achieved through systematically building knowledge, skills and competencies to give people more control at a local level.

## BOX 5.4: Health promotion and empowerment in Lofa County, Liberia

Lofa County was the epicentre for the Ebola outbreak in Liberia. This county is situated between Sierra Leone and Guinea, two neighbouring countries also experiencing Ebola, and many of the recorded cases were imported through the movement of people across the borders. To contain the further spread of the disease the local authorities decided to engage quickly with faith leaders and to establish community watch groups.

The involvement of youth and women were used as volunteer peer mobilisers and the cross-border monitoring of people's movement around the community was supervised by local cooperatives. The community imposed its own restrictions; for example, its members were not allowed to be involved in the burial of suspected or confirmed Ebola deaths. The community members were instead encouraged to use the 'Ebola hotlines' or to inform the district health officer of any community deaths. Community health volunteers were assigned for contact tracing in collaboration with local chiefs and district health officers. Agency guidelines for a safe and dignified burial were followed by the official burial teams with a special request from communities for the disinfection of affected households and personal effects.

Communities affected by Ebola were quickly reached with health messages and the distribution of hygiene kits. A combination of communication channels was used including interpersonal communication, posters and group discussions. Local businesses were also encouraged to collaborate by providing community radios for the promotion of the ongoing campaign 'No more Ebola in our Community!', through outreach activities. Testimonies from Ebola survivors were used to increase confidence in the affected communities, and Ebola hotspots were targeted for awareness raising by the volunteer mobilisers. Maintaining the motivation of health workers and volunteers was essential for the overall response and required robust team work and collaboration among partners.

The collaboration between the local authorities, response agencies and the communities was maintained through a consultative forum to support logistics, training, procurement and distribution of medical and non-medical supplies. The agencies provided transportation and additional human resource support for Ebola case investigation, contact tracing and the supervision of safe and dignified burials.

The response in the Lofa county was a collaborative approach in which the communities empowered themselves by gaining more control over everyday activities associated with the containment of the Ebola virus disease (Partners' Meeting Monrovia 2014). The local people acted at an individual, small group and partnership levels to effectively organise and mobilise the key stakeholders involved in the response.

## HEALTH ACTIVISM

Health activism involves a challenge to the existing order whenever it is perceived to influence peoples' health negatively or has led to an injustice or an inequity. What constitutes as activism depends on what is conventional in society as any action is relative to others used by individuals, groups and organisations. In practice, activist organisations use a combination of conventional and unconventional strategies to achieve their goals (Laverack 2013a). Health activism has an explicit purpose to help to empower others, and this is embodied in actions that are typically energetic, passionate, innovative and committed. The strategic approach used by activists is a dynamic process because organisations can use a variety of tactics that are culturally informed and to some extent shaped by local laws, political opportunity, culture and technology. The tactics of health activism also continue to evolve with new developments in technology; cell phone messaging, for example, is extensively used to organise public protests (Plows 2007).

> ## BOX 5.5: The Bhopal gas emergency, India
>
> The Bhopal gas emergency occurred between 2 and 3 December 1984 at the Union Carbide India Limited (UCIL) pesticide plant in India. A leak of methyl isocyanate gas and other chemicals resulted in the exposure of hundreds of thousands of people to toxic chemicals. The immediate death toll was 2259 people, and a government affidavit in 2006 stated the leak caused 558,125 injuries including 38,478 partially and approximately 3900 severely and permanently disabling injuries. UCIL was the Indian subsidiary of Union Carbide Corporation (UCC) in the United States. In June 2010, seven ex-employees, including the former UCIL chairman, were convicted in Bhopal of causing death by negligence and sentenced to imprisonment, the maximum punishment allowed by law. A group of Bhopal activists in America held a demonstration outside the Indian Embassy, demanding that the Indian Prime Minister provide justice to the Bhopal gas tragedy victims and extradite the then UCC chief to India. They held demonstrations in front of the Gandhi statue and submitted a petition to the Prime Minister of India through the embassy in the United States. The activists called their movement the 'International Campaign for Justice in Bhopal' and demanded for a cleaning up of the site in Bhopal and greater compensation to the victims affected by the tragedy (Oneindia 2010).

The types of actions that health activists typically engage in can be broadly sub-divided into two categories: indirect and direct.

1. Indirect actions are non-violent and often require a minimum of effort including voting, signing a petition, taking part in a 'virtual (on-line) sit-in' and sending an email to protest your cause.
2. Direct actions can range from peaceful protests to inflicting intentional physical damage to persons and property. For most activists, their focus is on short-term, reactive, direct action with the primary, and often only, means of a strategy being to have a real-time and immediate effect. Direct actions can be further sub-divided into non-violent and violent actions.
    a. Non-violent, direct actions include protests, picketing, vigils, marches, publicity campaigns and taking legal action.
    b. Direct violent actions include physical tactics against people or property and placing oneself in a position of manufactured vulnerability to prevent action or taking part in a civil disobedience.

Direct action can be used in a symbolic way to send a message to the general public; the owners, shareholders and employees of a specific company; or policy makers about specific grievances. Some organisations use a dual strategic approach which is moderate and conventional, while also using unconventional and more radical tactics. The radical strategy can be carried out by individuals or covert affinity groups, independent of the organisation, whereas the conventional tactics form its official actions. The dynamics of this relationship is often unclear, but a strategy that employs both tactics can have a dramatic influence on public opinion. The risk is that the unconventional tactics can result in negative publicity and impact on future resource allocation and recruitment (Martin 2007).

# 6

# The global Ebola virus disease response

## KEY POINTS

- The Ebola outbreak undermined already fragile national healthcare systems that were unprepared at almost every level to contain the disease.
- Local people must be fully involved in an outbreak response.
- Communities cannot intentionally empower themselves without first understanding the underlying causes of their powerlessness.
- Ebola preys on love for family and friends and leads to unsafe behaviours and resistance to efforts to change traditional practices.
- Community fears can be quickly alleviated when people are engaged and informed about the purpose of specific decisions.

The outbreak of the Ebola virus disease (EVD) in West Africa occurred between 2014 and 2016 and was the largest on record with an unprecedented number of reported cases ($n = 28,616$ at 9 August 2016) and deaths ($n = 11,310$ at 9 August 2016) (World Health Organization 2015c). The outbreak saw a rapid transmission of the disease within and across three countries: Guinea, Liberia, and Sierra Leone. The person-to-person mode of transmission also allowed the EVD to be spread through international travel to other countries such as to the United States. The imported cases provoked intense media coverage and public anxiety and heightened the reality of a risk to all countries. This ignited a global Ebola response although the disease never truly posed a global risk to public health.

> The Ebola outbreak undermined already fragile national healthcare systems that were unprepared at almost every level to contain the disease.

The three affected countries, which had never experienced an Ebola outbreak, were unprepared at almost every level, from early detection to delivering an appropriate response. Ebola outbreaks have occurred in Africa in the past, for example, in Equatorial Africa when the spread of the disease had mainly been through healthcare facilities (Hewlett and Hewlett 2008). However, in West Africa the Ebola virus outbreak behaved differently and was influenced by cultural and geographical influences and a weak surveillance system. Fear also became a cause of transmission of the disease as people left their homes, sometimes taking the Ebola virus with them to other settlements. The urban context also become a setting of transmission, including the capital cities of all three countries (Freetown, Monrovia and Conakry), which further increased concerns of an even more rapid spread of the disease in densely populated slum areas.

Several key factors have been identified as directly contributing to the rapid spread of the EVD in West Africa, including the health systems, healthcare workers and poor transportation services. This was exacerbated by a high degree of population movement across the porous borders of the three countries that created difficulties in contact tracing and led to patients seeking treatment elsewhere. Endemic infectious diseases including malaria, cholera and Lassa fever mimicked the early symptoms of Ebola. This complicated the process of diagnosis, contact tracing, care and treatment. Treatment by traditional healers was a preferred option for many people, and traditional customs and beliefs such as returning home to die, unsafe burial practices and secret societies increased the risk of disease transmission. Access to communities by agencies to help prevent the disease was inhibited by resistance caused by fear, rumour and professional malpractice. Early health messages emphasised that the disease was extremely serious and had no vaccine, treatment or cure. Although intended to promote protective behaviours these messages increased fear, rumour and resistance. The Ebola outbreak demonstrated the lack of international capacity to cooperate and to coordinate a collective response to a severe health emergency (World Health Organization 2015e).

The United Nations (UN) Secretary General officially launched the United Nations Mission for Ebola Emergency Response (UNMEER) on 19 September 2014. This followed the approval of a UN General Assembly resolution and UN Security Council resolution that declared the Ebola outbreak an international threat to peace and security. The main function of UNMEER was the coordination of the UN response to the EVD (Kamradt-Scott et al. 2015). The first priority in the West African outbreak was for sufficient beds for patients. This was soon met and the focus shifted to surveillance, case management, safe burials, contact tracing and to a lesser extent, social mobilisation. The largely top-down strategy was driven by the need to treat patients. However, the reported number of cases continued to increase and more severe measures began to follow, for example, in Sierra Leone on 19 September 2014 a 3-day stay-at-home 'lockdown' period was enforced, with the threat of fines or jail if violated. During this period, health promoters went door to door in search of people showing symptoms of infection, providing information and giving out resources and information leaflets. New cases of Ebola were identified and some communities were quarantined. People violated the quarantine requirements, and the government decided to implement a modified stay-at-home intervention in March 2015 which allowed more flexibility, for example, for people to attend prayers (Laverack and Manoncourt 2015).

## THE ROLE OF HEALTH PROMOTION IN PREVENTING THE SPREAD OF THE EBOLA VIRUS

Ebola control efforts must actively involve people and many agencies did learn from their earlier mistakes in the outbreak to make a genuine attempt to better engage with communities. The use of top-down tactics had a questionable effect, potentially worsening the epidemic and contributing to a greater social and economic burden (Institute of Development Studies 2015). During the Ebola response communities did understand what was required and did learn rapidly to change high-risk practices to help to reduce the transmission of the disease. In particular, community engagement can offer an added value through involvement in the management of quarantines, the control of cross-border movement, safe and dignified burials and the siting of Ebola Community Care Units.

> Local people must be fully involved in an outbreak response.

Health promotion made an important contribution to the outbreak because it enabled people to take more control over their lives and health. Community capacity building, participation and empowerment are intrinsic to a health promotion practice that recognises the value of a bottom-up approach. This provides real guidance to governments and agencies on how best to work with communities in future outbreaks. At the country level, the responsibility for communication and community engagement is usually with the health education or health promotion department of the Ministry of Health. This is also the official focal point for agencies involved in delivering communication services in the response.

At the local level, many community leaders recognised at an early stage the value of prevention as the best strategy to curtail the EVD. This included improved personal hygiene, surveillance, community-led quarantines and the management of cross-border movement. Chiefdoms in Kono, Sierra Leone, for example, wanted their own burial teams to counter the culturally insensitive handling of the dead by the local authorities. Others wanted community Ebola cemeteries where they could bury their dead, so future generations would have a referential ancestral burial site (Bah-Wakefield 2015). However, these measures were felt to be too risky for cross-infection by the authorities, so modified guidelines were used to provide safer and dignified burial procedures. Coercion, if subtly used by authorities, can be a useful procedure, but if not, it can be counterproductive. For example, there were negative repercussions of using forced quarantines by the military in Liberia, and this was responsible for a breaking down of community trust, an essential ingredient for the successful engagement of the local population in a response (ACAPS 2015).

## COMMUNITY-LED EBOLA ACTION

The Community-Led Ebola Action (CLEA) approach was developed by the Social Mobilisation Action Consortium, in conjunction with the Ministry of Health and Sanitation in Sierra Leone. The CLEA approach encourages the community to take responsibility and local actions to directly address an Ebola outbreak. It starts by enabling people to make their own appraisal and analysis of the Ebola outbreak and the likely future impacts if no action is taken. This helps to create a sense of urgency and a desire to develop a community action plan. Communities can decide how they will protect families; ensure safe and dignified burials; respond to sick people; utilise available health services; and create a supportive stigma-free environment for survivors, vulnerable children and others directly affected by the disease. The CLEA approach recognises that a bottom-up strategy can help to build trust between communities and authorities, for example, by listening to community concerns and considering their social and cultural needs. The CLEA approach ensures that communities have more of a voice in how the response is delivered and an ownership of specific actions that they can take to protect themselves. Importantly, this can be achieved without having to wait for external support and resources. At the community level the CLEA approach uses the following steps: (1) preparation, (2) triggering, (3) action planning and (4) follow-up (SMAC 2014). This approach could be adapted to other outbreak responses.

## Step 1. Preparation

The first step involves identifying and mapping issues, gaining permission to enter communities and planning events. The focus is on reaching those communities most affected and most at risk in emerging Ebola 'hotspots'. Strong, supportive leadership is often a critical success factor to inspire communities to take action. The amount of time and exposure to the EVD by the community can also greatly impact on its willingness to take action. Experience with CLEA has shown that a failure to consult with all stakeholders can lead to problems, especially with local chiefs and leaders at all levels of sub-national governance. The important aspects of the preparation are planning, engagement and consultation with the key stakeholders.

## Step 2. Triggering

The next step involves entering communities and building rapport, facilitating participatory analysis and supporting community action planning, if communities decide to make a plan. Triggering is about stimulating a collective sense of urgency to act in the face of the outbreak and to realise the consequences of inaction or of inappropriate action. The objectives are to (1) facilitate analysis so that community members can decide for themselves that the outbreak poses a real but preventable and treatable risk and (2) help communities gain clarity on available services and discuss how these services can be best suited to community needs. The community members then decide how to deal with the problem and to take action. The triggering point is the stage at which members of a community either decide to act together to prevent the spread of the disease or express doubts. Follow-up at this point is therefore critical to the success of the approach.

# Step 3. Action planning

It is very important that the community begins a discussion around the specific actions they want to work on involving the community members and to ensure that the leadership does not dominate the discussion. The community reflects on the previous discussions to recall whether there were any actions already mentioned and then on immediate actions to make positive changes. It is important to identify 'Community Champions' and to encourage them to take an active role in the action plans. Community Champions often emerge during the triggering process and may be women, men, youth, the elderly or people with special roles such as midwives. Community Champions are critical to success because they can follow-up with community members, who might be their neighbours, and encourage changes and the implementation of the agreed action plan. Community Champions will also be involved in Community Watch Committees, early reporting of cases, safe and dignified burials and supporting Ebola survivors. During this step the community may decide to form a 'community board' for supervising the implementation of the plan. This involves a small group that represents the different parts of the community such as women, youth and Ebola survivors. During action planning, the community board decides on how often they want to meet and who wants to lead on particular activities within a realistic time frame.

> Communities cannot intentionally empower themselves without first understanding the underlying causes of their powerlessness.

## STRATEGIC PLANNING FOR COLLECTIVE DECISION-MAKING

Community groups cannot intentionally empower themselves without having an understanding of the underlying causes of their situation, their strengths and their weaknesses. This understanding may occur slowly but can be facilitated through a process that promotes strategic planning for collective decision-making as follows: ranking key options, decision-making on the key actions to be taken, decision-making on the activities for the key actions to be taken and an identification of resources (Laverack 2015).

## RANKING KEY OPTIONS

The group of representatives first makes a list of the key options covering the particular health concern, for example, how to prevent the spread of the EVD in their community. The health promoter can help by providing specific technical information about the causes of disease transmission and by helping the participants to rank their concerns; for example, that infected body fluids entering another person's body can cause the transmission of the disease, a simple principle that has to be equally understood by both the health promoter and the recipients of the message. The ranking must come from the group without being coerced by the health promoter. If the number of ranked options is large, the health promoter can assist the group to produce a prioritised list and this might include the following:

- To avoid physical contact with a sick person, his or her body fluids and objects used while sick with Ebola
- To increase hand-washing
- To report suspected cases to the authorities
- To stop unknown people entering the community

A prioritised list of the different choices is in itself insufficient to help others to empower themselves. This information must also be transformed into actions and this is achieved through decisions about positive changes.

## DECISION-MAKING ON THE KEY ACTIONS TO BE TAKEN

The group is next asked to decide on how the situation can be improved for each ranked issue. The purpose is to first identify the most feasible actions that will improve the present situation and then to provide a more detailed strategy outlining the activities. Taking the first prioritised health option – to avoid physical contact with a sick person, his or her body fluids and objects used while sick with Ebola – the decisions on the key actions to be taken might include the following:

- To identify a place where the suspected case can safely stay
- To ask authorities to disinfect and remove objects owned by the case
- To provide a supply of food and water for the suspected case
- To provide a list of people who were in contact with the suspected case of Ebola
- To provide a list of people who will act as a contact between the sick person and his or her family

## DECISIONS ON THE KEY ACTIVITIES FOR EACH ACTION TAKEN

The group is next asked to consider in practice the most feasible actions that can be carried out and, in particular, to sequence activities to make an improvement and to set a realistic time frame. Continuing from the example above, the activities to implement the identified actions and might include the following:

- Get permission to use the place where the suspected case can stay
- Make sure the place is empty and clean and ready to use
- Collect money to buy food for the sick person
- Identify a safe place to store the food

## IDENTIFICATION OF RESOURCES

The group next identifies the resources that are necessary to implement the actions they have identified. The health promoter can help to map the necessary resources to undertake the actions and might include the following:

- Money to buy food, bedding, etc.
- People available to act as helpers

- Advice on how to prevent transmission of the disease from the health promoter
- Money to pay for transport if the person has to be taken to a treatment centre

## THE DECISION-MAKING MATRIX

The matrix provides a summary of the decisions and actions to be undertaken and is the basis for an 'informal contract' between the health promoter and the community members. It identifies specific tasks or responsibilities usually set against a time frame. It also identifies the resources that will be required to fulfil these tasks and responsibilities, within the agreed time frame, by both the health promoter and the community members.

| Priority | Key decisions | Key activities | Resources |
|---|---|---|---|
| • To avoid physical contact with a sick person, his or her body fluids and objects they used while sick with Ebola | • To identify a place where the suspected case can safely stay<br>• To ask authorities to disinfect and remove objects owned by the case<br>• To provide a supply of food and water for the suspected case<br>• To provide a list of people who were in contact with the suspected case of Ebola<br>• To provide a list of people who will act as a contact between the sick person and his or her family | • Get permission to use the place where the suspected case can stay<br>• Make sure the place is empty and clean and ready to use<br>• Collect money to buy food for the sick person<br>• Identify a safe place to store the food | • Money to buy food, bedding, etc.<br>• People available to act as helpers<br>• Advice on how to prevent transmission of the disease from the health promoter<br>• Money to pay for transport if the person has to be taken to a treatment centre |

# Step 4. Follow-up

The final step involves supporting and encouraging communities to implement their action plans and sharing up-to-date information about available health services. The format of the follow-up can include regular phone calls and household visits and also support to Community Champions and local community boards. The health promoter can begin to support the momentum in communities that have already developed an action plan and who have begun to mobilise local people.

The flow of money between an agency and communities is an important and subtle follow-up consideration that must be handled carefully. The following are examples of sociocultural factors that were taken from the West African Ebola response:

- Resources are often distributed informally, for example, cell phone credit or motorbike fuel.
- Paying cash can be seen as opening an ongoing relationship of goods and services and not just a one-off payment.
- At an individual and household level, many people find it difficult to save as they are in a continual state of debt to others in their neighbourhood. Receiving goods on credit is therefore normal behaviour.
- Communities have developed various mechanisms to save money, for example, 'esusu' schemes involving money circulated by a group of people adding a specific amount on a regular basis and using it as an emergency fund.
- The major daily household expenditure is food and is managed by women.
- 'Ebola money' can have both a positive and negative impact at the household level by creating tension between household members.
- Financial payments can become 'hijacked' by specific individuals in the community such as local leaders who then do not distribute it equitably. This raises issues about the fair and accountable distribution of finances.
- Existing social networks and non-government organisations can be used to quickly distribute financial incentives (Bedford 2014).

## THE ROLE OF HEALTH PROMOTION IN SAFE AND DIGNIFIED BURIALS

The World Health Organization has developed guidelines for the safe and dignified management of the burial of patients who have died from suspected or confirmed EVD (World Health Organization 2015). The 12 steps identify the different stages that burial teams have to follow and start before the burial teams arrive in the village up to their return to the operational headquarters. The 12 steps are as follows: Step 1. Before departure: team composition and preparation of disinfectants; Step 2. Assemble all necessary equipment; Step 3. Arrival at deceased patient home: prepare burial with family and evaluate risks; Step 4. Put on all personal protective equipment (PPE); Step 5. Placement of the body in the body bag; Step 6. Placement of the body bag in a coffin where culturally appropriate; Step 7. Sanitise family's environment; Step 8. Remove PPE, manage waste and perform hand hygiene; Step 9. Transport the coffin or the body bag to the cemetery; Step 10. Burial at the cemetery: place coffin or body bag into the grave; Step 11. Burial at the cemetery: engaging community for prayers; and Step 12. Return to the hospital or team headquarters.

Several of the steps in the approach have a specific role for health promotion including community engagement, awareness raising, training, assessing community perceptions and ensuring that the cultural practices and beliefs are respected.

## Assemble all necessary equipment

Burial bags are assembled to hold the body of the deceased and to safely contain blood and body fluids. Equipment to prevent infections such as alcohol-based solutions, soap and towels or chlorine solution, PPE and disposable gloves are prepared. The colour of the body bags can assist with a dignified burial because white is often associated with death and this means that a white body bag can act as a shroud without the need to further prepare the body (see Shrouding procedure below). However, this information was processed too late by some international agencies that had already supplied, in large quantities, black body bags. Health promoters are available to explain the use of the body bags and, when

---

**BOX 6.1: The demonstration of Personal Protective Equipment**

Members of the burial teams and staff at the Ebola treatment centres use personal protective equipment (PPE), and community members have raised concerns about their appearance and behaviour. The exercise helps to dispel some of the myths and fears surrounding the use of PPE. For example, communities may see the PPE as further proof that intruders arriving dressed in PPE are associated with sorcery. The purpose is to demonstrate what each piece of PPE is for and why it is important in preventing the transmission of the Ebola virus. Community members will be able to touch and feel the PPE and to discuss ways it could be made less fearful. The exercise takes about 30 minutes.

1. Take the sample PPE and spread the pieces of the suit out on the ground.
2. Invite people to take a look at these items. Encourage them to touch them and pick them up. Do not force anyone to touch the suit if they do not want to.
3. A volunteer will demonstrate how the PPE, including the suit, boots, eye protection, facemask and gloves, is put on and worn.
4. Throughout the demonstration, encourage questions and discussion, for example, when and why it should be worn and how to dispose of it safely.
5. When the demonstration is finished, encourage community members to offer ideas on how to make the experience of interacting with teams in PPE less fearful (SMAC 2014).

possible, to accommodate the cultural needs of the family. Health promoters can also provide training in the proper use of PPE.

## Arrival at the deceased patient home: Prepare burial with family and evaluate risks

In practice the burial teams can arrive with vehicles and equipment at a household without giving the family enough time to grieve or to accept the situation. A health promoter may be able to arrive in advance to meet with the family and community leaders, explain the process and the reasons for the process and then ask permission for the rest of the team to come for the burial. This can help to reduce community resistance and ensures a more respectful burial. As another way to avoid anxiety in the community, the team should not be wearing PPE upon arrival. Greet the family and offer condolences before unloading the necessary materials. The health promoter should contact a local faith representative at the request of the family members to arrange to meet at the place of collection for the burial of the deceased. If a local faith representative is not available the health promoter can use a list of phone contacts, with the agreement of the family. The health promoter and the faith representative should work together with the family witness (such as a paternal uncle) to make sure that the burial is carried out in a dignified manner. The burial team waits while the faith representative and family witness can be called and have completed their discussion with the health promoter about the safe and dignified burial. Family members are identified who will be participating in the burial rituals (prayers, orations, closing of the coffin). If the family has prepared a coffin, they may wish to carry it to the place of burial. The grave should already be prepared, if this is not the case, selected people should be sent to dig the grave at the area identified by the family. Family members witness the preparation activities of the body of the deceased patient and are asked for any specific requests, for example, about what to do with the personal effects of the deceased (burn, bury in the grave or disinfect). The family witness and family members can take pictures of the preparation and burial and may want to prepare a civil, cultural or religious item, for example, an identity plaque, cross or picture of deceased, for the identification of the grave.

> Ebola preys on love for family and friends and leads to unsafe behaviours and resistance to efforts to change traditional practices.

Faith-based groups play a key role in disseminating information and helping to mobilise communities to undertake preventive measures and to support bereaved families and survivors. The percentages of the Muslim population in, for example, Sierra Leone (77%) and Guinea (85%) are significant as are Christian and animist beliefs. However, traditional beliefs were not always respected or could not be accommodated; for example, in the Muslim tradition the dead should be buried before sundown; however, during Ebola over-stretched government burial teams sometimes arrived days after a death. The boxes below provide specific sociocultural requirements for a dignified burial with both Christian and Muslim patients.

---

**BOX 6.2: Procedure for the dignified burial of a Christian patient**

Specific requirements for the dignified burial of a Christian patient include the following:

- Giving the family the opportunity to view as an and an alternative to touching and bathing the body, for example, sprinkling of water over the body or reading a scripture, placing the written scripture verse on the body before closing the body bag.
- Provide a symbol of dignity and clothing.
- Identify a religious leader known or accepted by the family. The priest can offer spiritual consolation, can pray with the family and can read appropriate scriptures.
- Identify a burial site the family can accept and ensure the grave is appropriately labelled.
- Allow the family members the opportunity to be involved in the digging or preparation of the grave, if that is their custom or preference.
- Once the body or coffin is in the grave, allow the family members the option to throw the first soil in or on the grave according to local practice, hierarchy or tradition.
- Allow the family to prepare or place the label or religious symbol at the grave, for example, a cross. A memorial service can be held at a later date, as per custom or preference.

---

**BOX 6.3: Procedure for the dignified burial of a Muslim patient**

**DRY ABLUTION**

This procedure should only be carried out by a Muslim person or Muslim faith representative once the deceased has been placed in the body bag. A short Arabic prayer of intention is said over the deceased. The person carrying out the dry ablution, such as the Muslim Burial team member (in personal protective equipment [PPE]), softly strikes his or her hands on clean sand or stone and then gently passes over the hands and then the face of the deceased. This represents the ablution that would normally have been done with water. A short Arabic prayer is said over the deceased. The body bag is closed if no request for shrouding has been made. This simple procedure only takes about 1–2 minutes.

> **SHROUDING**
>
> A plain unstitched white cotton sheet (scented with musk, camphor or perfumed) is placed on top of the opened body bag. The deceased is lifted by the Burial team (in PPE) and placed on top of the shroud. The extended side edges of the shroud are pulled over the top of the deceased to cover the head, body, legs and feet. Three strips cut from the same fabric are used to tie and close up the shroud: one for above the head, one for below the feet and one for around the middle of the body. It is knotted at both ends. If there is a female member of the burial team, she should shroud the deceased female patients. The body bag is closed.

## Sanitise the environment

Disinfect any body fluids and gather in a plastic bag bed linen, clothes and objects of the deceased that were not placed in the coffin and need to be buried with the coffin. Straw mats soiled with body fluid of the deceased patient should be burnt at a distance from the house. The health promoter should explain this procedure to the family and ensure they have given permission to destroy these items.

## Transport the coffin or the body bag to the cemetery

Distribute household gloves to the family members who will carry the coffin. Respect the time of grieving, possibly with a speech about the deceased and religious songs (chants) to aid the departure of the deceased to the cemetery, according to cultural and religious practices. The expression of pain and loss through shouting, crying and songs should be respected by the burial team. The health promoter should ensure that customs and rituals are respected, for example, to allow time for people to express their feelings.

## Burial at the cemetery: Place coffin or body bag into the grave

Manually carry the coffin or body bag to the grave followed by the funeral participants. Place the coffin or body bag clothes and objects belonging to the deceased into the grave. The health promoter should ensure that customs and rituals are respected, for example, to allow for the spirit of the deceased to be liberated. Burial rites have spiritual connotations and if people are prevented from washing, touching or kissing the dead, it can be perceived as endangering the family and can have a psychological effect on the whole community (Bah 2015). However, this type of a situation can be reconciled; for example, an Ebola outbreak in the Democratic Republic of Congo in 2014 was quickly contained because community elders were given control over decisions about making traditional practices safer (Heymann 2015).

# Burial at the cemetery: Engaging the community for prayers

The health promoter should take the lead in engaging the community for prayers as this helps to dissipate tension. Respect should be given for the time required for prayers and funeral speeches to be carried out. Family members and their assistants should be allowed to place an identification (name of the deceased and the date) on the grave and a religious symbol if requested. The burial team should attend the funeral and offer condolences, for example, by signing the condolences book. The family may communally wash hands with disinfectant after the burial as a sign of commitment to help prevent the spread of Ebola.

# THE ROLE OF HEALTH PROMOTION IN EBOLA COMMUNITY CARE UNITS

Ebola treatment units are purpose-built, professionally run and medically staffed centres for the treatment and care of Ebola cases. However, the rapid transmission of the disease resulted in the need to provide temporary treatment units to ensure that sufficient facilities were available. This is an extreme measure that could occur in many communicable disease outbreaks. An Ebola Community Care Unit (ECCU) is a temporarily constructed facility of 8–10 beds where infected patients can be moved to be isolated and yet still receive basic care supported by health workers and members of their family. The ECCU is usually located close to the community and serves as the first point of isolation while people are waiting for referral to an Ebola treatment unit. It is crucial to involve the community in the siting, planning, construction and running of the ECCU, with support from health workers. Admission to an ECCU can increase the chances of a person's survival and can interrupt any further transmission of the disease among the family and community. However, care must be taken because the makeshift nature of the ECCU can place caregivers and healthcare workers at an increased risk; may promote the unsafe transport of sick persons; and can use inadequate procedures, for example, for the safe disposal of waste materials.

The example below follows the process used by the Sierra Leone Emergency Management Programme to establish Ebola Community Care Units (Sierra Leone Emergency Management Programme 2014) and explains the role of health promotion.

> Community fears can be quickly alleviated when people are engaged and informed about the purpose of specific decisions.

# Community engagement and ECCUs

A coordinated approach that can be easily understood by all stakeholders is essential in any strategy for community engagement. Standard operating procedures are also useful to help establish community engagement prerequisites and a systematic approach that will allow personnel and services to be delivered to the ECCU, at the request of the community, with its full understanding and participation. Health promotion has an important role in engaging with communities in regard to the construction and use of ECCUs and in providing updated information about the progression of the outbreak and the availability of available services. The health promoter works in cooperation with the national government to encourage participation during the management of the ECCU. This is especially important in areas of intense and widespread transmission and where community resistance may hinder the role of health workers. For example, a rapid assessment of the siting and construction of ECCU in Sierra Leone found that the fears of communities were quickly alleviated when they had been actively engaged and informed about the decision-making process (ICAP 2015) (Figure 6.1).

The strategic approach to encourage community participation in the establishment of an ECCU can be achieved in three phases: planning, operational and exit.

## ECCU PLANNING PHASE

The ECCU planning phase indicates that community engagement has not yet been achieved. Personnel other than the neighbourhood support team should not enter or approach the community until this phase has been completed. This phase begins with an orientation and sensitisation of the District Health Management Team. The key health promotion messages include the scope of services and duration of the ECCU, roles and responsibilities and the identification of the Community Engagement and Mobilization Team (CEMT). The CEMT organises mobilisation meetings at chiefdom levels under the leadership of the Paramount Chief. Councillors, community elders, religious leaders, teachers, women and youth representatives participate in the meetings. Key messages

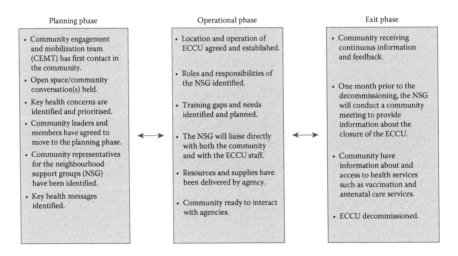

Figure 6.1 Engaging communities and Ebola community care units.

are the identification of a neighbourhood support group (NSG) linked to each ECCU, skills training and how the NSG will act as a bridge between the community and health staff at the ECCU to address any ongoing issues that arise during the strategy. The NSG organises an open-space community dialogue to give people an opportunity to voice their feelings, ask questions and identify what they feel are the most important health issues in their locality.

## ECCU OPERATIONAL PHASE

The ECCU operational phase indicates that the ECCU has been established and is operational in agreement with the community representatives. During the operational phase, the overall guidance and support of a coordinating agency such as a non-government organisation will help the NSG to conduct communication activities within communities through house-to-house visits and with identified community and religious leaders. The NSG will facilitate contact tracing by preventing non-compliant behaviour including threats and protests. The NSG will mobilise people and households that develop symptoms of Ebola to go to the ECCU and will organise hand-washing facilities and help coordinate safe burials. The NSG will liaise directly with both the community and with the ECCU staff.

## ECCU EXIT PHASE

The ECCU exit phase indicates that the community representatives have agreed to allow other personnel into or near to the community to prevent and control the transmission of the disease. The community is continually informed by the health promoter about the scope of services and duration of the operation of the ECCU to help with local expectations. After the declaration of the end of the outbreak the ECCU is usually decommissioned. With the assistance of the health promoter, 1 month before the decommissioning, the NSG will conduct a community meeting to provide information about the closure of the ECCU. During house-to-house visits the NSG will also promote the use of other health services such as vaccination and antenatal care services (Sierra Leone Emergency Management Program 2014).

# 7

# Health promotion and person-to-person disease outbreaks

---

| **KEY POINTS** |
|---|
| • Health promotion in person-to-person disease transmission can help people to protect themselves through simple behaviour changes. |
| • Raising awareness of hygiene practices such as hand-washing with soap after contact with human faeces can be an effective intervention with large health benefits. |
| • Being involved with groups enables individuals to become better organised and mobilised towards collectively addressing their needs. |
| • Targeting the uptake of vaccination can be an effective approach with large health benefits in some disease outbreaks. |
| • The use of commonly available technology such as mobile phones can be an effective channel of communication to raise awareness levels. |

A communicable disease is transmitted from a source, such as from a person, and can be prevented by using interventions that focus on controlling or eliminating the route of transmission. Communicable diseases that can be transmitted from one person to another person include the poliovirus, cholera, Middle East respiratory syndrome (MERS), severe acute respiratory syndrome (SARS), tuberculosis and sexually transmitted diseases. Health promotion helps to prevent disease transmission by enabling people to understand how to protect themselves and their communities through simple behaviour changes such as hand-washing; condom use; modification of the social or physical environment, or both; and vaccination to reduce the effect of the disease (Public Health Agency of Canada 2013).

> Health promotion in person–to-person disease transmission can help people to protect themselves from through simple behaviour changes.

In this chapter I address the role of health promotion in person-to-person disease transmission through examples of outbreak responses. First, for potentially the next global outbreak, avian influenza, followed by a focus on cholera, a disease closely linked to health emergencies; global eradication of the poliovirus; and MERS, a disease often transmitted in healthcare facilities.

## AVIAN INFLUENZA

The Ebola virus was the first disease to be declared a global security threat by the United Nations, but what infectious agent will cause the next international health emergency? This will possibly be an airborne virus that can be rapidly transmitted person to person, has a high mortality ratio and that has migrated into the human population from a zoonotic source such as domesticated animals. Avian influenza outbreaks are unpredictable but occur when key factors converge, including a zoonotic virus with the ability to cause sustained person-to-person transmission to which the population has little or no immunity. With the growth of global trade and travel, a localised outbreak can rapidly transform into a pandemic with little time to develop a vaccine or to prepare a global public health response.

Creating a candidate vaccine virus (CVV) would be a first step and is an influenza virus that can be used by manufacturers to produce a flu vaccine. In addition to preparing CVVs for seasonal flu vaccine production, they can also be developed for novel avian influenza (bird flu) viruses with pandemic potential as part of preparedness activities. Data collected through global and animal flu surveillance informs the selection of CVVs, and experts choose CVVs against wild-type viruses in nature that pose a risk to human health. The creation of a CVV is a multi-step process that takes about 2 months for a novel avian influenza, usually longer than for creating a seasonal flu CVV (Centers for Disease Control and Prevention 2017). This creates a period during which the virus can spread internationally; and even when available, low vaccine stocks might limit coverage to only those who are most at risk such as healthcare workers. Super-spreading may also play an important role in transmission and high mortality levels at the beginning of an avian influenza outbreak (National Health Service 2017).

Avian influenza subtypes in poultry including A(H5) or A(H7N9) viruses are of a particular public health concern as they can cause severe illness in people and have the potential to mutate to become easily transmissible person to person. In particular, people can be infected with avian influenza virus subtypes A(H5N1), A(H7N9) and A(H9N2). Influenza type A viruses are classified into subtypes according to the combinations of different virus surface proteins haemagglutinin (H) and neuraminidase (N). Depending on the host, influenza A can be classified as avian influenza, swine influenza or as other types of animal influenza viruses. For example, 'bird flu' virus subtypes A(H5N1) and A(H9N2)

BOX 7.1: The 1918 Spanish flu pandemic

The 1918 Spanish flu pandemic (January 1918–December 1920) was an unusually deadly influenza outbreak involving the H1N1 virus and infecting an estimated 500 million people. The actual mortality rate of the pandemic is not known but is conservatively estimated at 10%–20% of those who were infected. This case–fatality ratio gives 3%–6% of the entire global population or as many as 40–50 million people died worldwide. A spike occurred in 1918 when the second wave occurred that had an even higher mortality rate. The first wave had resembled other typical flu epidemics when those most at risk were the sick and elderly. But in August 1918 the second wave began in France, Sierra Leone, and the United States, and an unusual feature of the outbreak was that it disproportionately killed healthy young adults. The explanations for the high mortality of the 1918 influenza pandemic include that the specific variant of the virus had an unusual aggressive nature, malnourishment, overcrowded hospitals, poor hygiene and possibly the existence of superspreaders. It remains unknown whether there was an animal-host origin of the pandemic virus and why the pandemic eventually died out after 18 months in summer 1919 (Johnson 2006).

or 'swine flu' virus subtypes A(H1N1) and A(H3N2). For human infections with the A(H7N9) virus the incubation period ranges from 1 to 10 days, with an average of 5 days and is longer than that for seasonal influenza at 2 days. The majority of human cases are from A(H5N1) and A(H7N9) infection that have been associated with direct or indirect contact with infected live or dead poultry. The viruses do not presently transmit easily from person to person, and sustained transmission has not yet been established. Some infections in people have been very severe, even resulting in deaths, but many infections have been mild in humans.

BOX 7.2: Human infection with avian influenza A(H7N9) in China

On 4 February 2017 the Centers for Disease Control and Prevention reported a laboratory-confirmed case of human infection with the avian influenza A(H7N9) virus. The patient, a 69-year-old male, travelled to Yangjiang City, Guangdong Province, China, and developed fever and chills on 23 January 2017. On 25 January 2017, the patient returned to Taiwan and visited the local hospital. During the medical consultation, neither fever nor pneumonia was detected and a rapid test for influenza on an oropharyngeal sample was negative. PCR testing of additional samples was obtained the next day and also tested negative for avian influenza A.

On 1 February 2017 the man again visited the hospital with a fever, cough and dyspnoea. Bilateral pneumonia was diagnosed, and the next day additional sputum samples were collected and were found to be positive for avian influenza A(H7N9) virus. No source of exposure to the avian influenza A(H7N9) virus was identified (World Health Organization 2017).

Antiviral drugs, notably oseltamivir (Tamiflu), can improve the prospects of survival of avian influenza. It is advised that in suspected cases, oseltamivir should be prescribed as soon as possible to maximise its therapeutic benefits and be considered in patients presenting later in the course of illness (World Health Organization 2017a). Other drugs under development include zanamivir and peramivir for intravenous use and favipiravir for oral use.

## HEALTH PROMOTION AND AVIAN INFLUENZA

Most human cases of avian influenza are transmitted through contact with infected poultry or contaminated environments such as live poultry markets and farms. Slaughtering and preparing poultry for consumption, including in household settings, are also risk factors for disease transmission. Infected birds transmit the virus in their saliva, mucous and faeces. People who work directly with poultry during an outbreak are at a high risk of transmission and should be the target for health promotion interventions. Person-to-person infections normally happen when the virus gets into the eyes, nose or mouth, or is inhaled in droplets or dust. Health promotion also has a role to target the general population to raise awareness about prevention practices such as hand-washing and about the early signs and symptoms of the disease. Health promotion can improve personal skills for infection control practices such as disinfection and can raise awareness about the effectiveness and availability of antiviral drugs. Everyone must be reminded of their responsibility to report suspected cases to the health authorities and can be facilitated through information about websites and emergency telephone numbers. Health promotion uses communication approaches to raise awareness, including the mass media, print materials and peer- or face-to-face education.

In health promotion messaging it is essential to explain why as well as what is necessary to help people understand the reason for the prescribed advice.

### People who work directly with poultry during an outbreak

The HPAI A(H5N1) virus has become entrenched in domestic poultry populations. Outbreaks have resulted in millions of poultry infections, several hundred human cases and many deaths. The health promotion advice during an outbreak of avian influenza has been to avoid poultry farms, avoid contact with animals in live bird markets, avoid entering areas where poultry may be slaughtered, and avoid contact with any surfaces that seem to be contaminated with faeces from poultry (World Health Organization 2017a). Controlling the circulation of avian influenza viruses in the poultry population is essential to reducing the risk of human infection and requires strong coordination between animal and public health authorities. Prevention zones can be put in place to reduce the threat to poultry from avian influenza. They require poultry keepers to take a variety of biosecurity precautions such as keeping poultry housed and increasing hygiene practices. Otherwise, the people who work with poultry or who respond to avian influenza outbreaks and are at a higher risk of infection are advised through health promotion to follow specific infection control practices, as follows:

- Regular hand-washing with warm water and soap
- Wear appropriate personal protective equipment including protective clothing, heavy gloves and boots, goggles and masks and receive adequate training on putting on, taking off and the hygienic disposal and disinfection of equipment
- Disinfection and disposal of contaminated personal clothing and other personal articles
- Monitor body temperature twice daily for fever and be aware of influenza-like symptoms
- Report to health authorities any symptoms and refer for diagnostic testing and treatment to reduce the severity of the disease (Centers for Disease Control and Prevention 2017)

People working directly with poultry in an outbreak response should receive seasonal influenza vaccination and take prophylactic antiviral medication during an outbreak. The seasonal influenza vaccine will not prevent infection with avian influenza A, but it can reduce the risk of co-infection with humans.

## The general population and the transmission of avian influenza

Although person-to-person transmission of avian influenza is presently low, except examples in small clusters reported among healthcare workers, the threat of a global outbreak is real (World Health Organization 2017a). Health promotion messaging for the general population is intended to help people to avoid infection, reduce the transmission of the disease and be vigilant in reporting suspected cases. This is achieved through increasing knowledge levels and providing personal skills for improved protection measures. People in the general population are advised to use the following prevention and control practices:

- Turn away from other people and cover your mouth with tissues when you cough or sneeze
- Dispose of tissues immediately after use and wash your hands with soap and warm water
- Avoid public places if you have symptoms

- Do not go near sick or dead birds
- Keep away from bird droppings and wash your hands thoroughly if you touch any droppings
- Avoid live animal markets or poultry farms
- As a precaution, always ensure good hygiene standards when preparing and cooking poultry; for example, use different utensils for cooked and raw poultry and wash your hands thoroughly with soap and warm water before and after handling poultry (Centers for Disease Control and Prevention 2017).

The international concern is that avian influenza will adapt quickly by acquiring genes from human viruses and then trigger one or more pandemics. The probability that an avian or another zoonotic influenza virus will result in a pandemic in the next few decades necessitates ongoing surveillance in both animal and human populations. Avian and other zoonotic influenza viruses are presently monitored through the Global Influenza Surveillance and Response System involving a collaboration between the World Health Organization (WHO), the World Organisation for Animal Health and the Food and Agriculture Organization of the United Nations to track and assess the risk from avian and other zoonotic influenza viruses to public health.

## CHOLERA OUTBREAKS

During 2013, 129,064 cases of cholera in total were notified from 47 countries, including 2102 deaths, and it is estimated that there are between 1.4 and 4.3 million un-notified cases and up to 142,000 un-notified deaths every year (Ali et al. 2012). The main reservoirs of cholera are people, and this acute diarrhoeal infection is caused by the ingestion of food or water contaminated with the bacterium *Vibrio cholerae*. The short incubation period of 2 hours to 5 days is a key factor that triggers the potentially rapid pattern of cholera outbreaks. About 80% of people infected with cholera do not develop any symptoms, although the bacteria are present in their faeces for 1–10 days after infection and are shed back into the environment, potentially infecting other people. Under the International Health Regulations the notification of cholera cases is not mandatory and countries do not require proof of cholera vaccination. An oral cholera vaccine stockpile was formally established in 2013 for outbreak control on the principle that vaccination does have a role in the prevention of cholera when it is used in conjunction with accessible healthcare and improvements in water supply, sanitation and hygiene promotion (World Health Organization 2015a).

### Cholera preparedness

Cholera preparedness and action plans are developed during the pre-outbreak phase. The start of a cholera outbreak can be identified by specific criteria; for example, the World Health Organization threshold is a 1% mortality (for every 1000 people at least 10 deaths). Other agencies use a more focused response in endemic areas, such as 0.6% mortality; or if the number of diarrhoea cases treated at clinics is constant but the number of deaths increase this can suggest that cholera is responsible. Likewise, if child mortality is caused by severe dehydration, this could also be an early indicator. These signs along with the testing of rectal swabs can help in the identification of a cholera outbreak.

A cholera outbreak response begins with identifying high-risk 'hotspots' to reduce the spread of the disease. Other measures include improving water supplies and sanitation, safe burial practices and controlling hygiene practices in communal gathering places such as markets. Community engagement and cholera-focused hygiene promotion can support the initial control measures in addition to surveillance and treatment. The response should be linked with ongoing country health programming that may require building local capacity to manage activities and strengthening the government departments that are responsible for essential services such as water supply and environmental health.

## HEALTH PROMOTION AND CHOLERA OUTBREAKS

Cholera is best prevented through the provision of safe water and sanitation. Hygiene promotion campaigns are also important to prevent the disease by targeting hand-washing with soap, the safe preparation and storage of food and breastfeeding. Infrastructural interventions to improve environmental conditions in conjunction with health and hygiene promotion include the development of piped water systems with water treatment facilities; interventions at the household level such as water filtration, water chemical or solar disinfection; safe water

### BOX 7.3: A cholera outbreak in the Central African Republic

A cholera outbreak was declared on 10 August 2016, with 46 confirmed cases and 13 deaths in the Central African Republic. The outbreak was the consequence of a civil crisis that had disrupted water and sanitation systems and had displaced a large proportion of the population into overcrowded areas. These insanitary and overcrowded conditions increase the risk of cholera transmission should the bacteria be present or introduced by the population. The reported cases were mainly from villages along the Oubangui River where the first case occurred after travelling from the neighbouring country of the Democratic Republic of Congo. In response, international agencies and the Ministry of Health and Sanitation activated a cholera control command centre with taskforces covering case management, surveillance, Water, Sanitation & Hygiene (WASH), risk communication and social mobilisation, security and safe burials. Patients were taken to a cholera treatment centre as well as ongoing water source treatment and community engagement activities in villages along the Oubangui River. However, the civil crisis made disease surveillance and healthcare delivery difficult in an already fragile public health system (World Health Organization 2016g).

storage containers; and the construction of systems for sewage disposal including private and public latrines.

> Raising awareness of hygiene practices such as hand-washing with soap after contact with human faeces can be an effective intervention with large health benefits.

## Hygiene promotion

Hygiene promotion aims to prevent communicable diseases, especially diarrhoeal diseases, through the widespread adoption of safe hygiene behaviours and improvements in environmental conditions (Appleton and Sijbesma 2005). Good hygiene practices are theoretically capable of reducing the infection with pathogens transmitted by the faecal–oral route. In particular, simple measures such as hand-washing with soap after contact with faeces represent acceptable behaviour change interventions with large health benefits (Curtis et al. 2001). Hygiene promotion starts with rapid data collection to find out and understand what different groups of people know about hygiene, what they do and what they want and why. These findings are used to design messages and implement activities that enable the different groups to reduce high-risk conditions and strengthen positive behaviours (UNICEF 1999).

### BOX 7.4: Preventing cholera transmission at funerals

In West Papua it is a traditional practice for the attendees of funerals to touch the dead body and then to feast afterward. People come long distances to attend burials, which may bring people from uninfected areas into contact with a cholera outbreak. They may then carry cholera back to their home villages and can spread the disease very fast over a wide area. Preventive measures at funerals focus on proper disinfection and engaging with key community and religious leaders to find ways of reducing the risks of the ceremony without damaging its cultural significance. In West Papua, religious leaders promoted proper hand-washing after people touch the corpse. Because this innovation did not undermine the significance of the ceremonies, the religious authorities were also quick to adopt this practice with the celebrants and to issue hygiene kits including soap, water treatment tablets and hand-washing buckets to help ensure that people followed proper hygiene procedures (Lamond and Kinjanyui 2012).

Participatory Hygiene and Sanitation Transformation (PHAST) and Self-esteem, Associative strength, Resourcefulness, Action planning, Responsibility (SARAR) are advanced hygiene approaches based on a set of participatory techniques to promote positive behaviours, improvements in water and sanitation and community management these facilities. Water, Sanitation & Hygiene (WASH) is a concept that groups together water, sanitation and hygiene to provide complementary strategies that have a greater impact in disease outbreak responses (International Red Cross 2013).

---

**BOX 7.5: Preventing cholera through schools**

In the Oromia region of Ethiopia, international response agencies were able to reach thousands of people with cholera prevention messages through schools and religious leaders within a short period. Health and Red Cross clubs (one per school) and religious leaders (two per village) were given 2 days of training to help pass messages onto their students and congregations. Some schools even closed and then sent their pupils to undertake outreach work. The schools set up a central information board, where cholera cases were recorded and the health centre was able to use these data for selecting targeted areas especially in remote communities (Lamond and Kinjanyui 2012).

---

Key hygiene messages for preventing cholera are developed using formative research and rapid assessment techniques as described in Chapter 2. However, the following messages provide key information that has been covered in a previous cholera outbreak response. It is essential to explain why as well as what is the best advice to help people understand the reason for the prescribed action:

1. Before drinking water, treat it. Chlorinate water. Store drinking water in clean and covered containers after treatment. **Note:** Boiling water should only be promoted as an option where it is feasible and done properly; that is water should be brought to a rolling boil, cooled and stored in clean containers before use.
2. Clean your hands. Rub off dirt from both hands. If you have soap and water, use it and wash by rubbing both of your hands. If soap is not available, rub dirt off using water and ash, sand, leaves or other locally materials. **Note:** Rubbing with the aid of a cleansing agent is most important. When? Before you eat or put anything into your mouth; after helping someone with symptoms, or cleaning up their excreta or vomit; before you prepare food; after cleaning a child's bottom and after defecating or visiting the toilet.
3. If someone is sick with cholera, replace liquid lost in diarrhoea or vomit by giving them a drink after every diarrhoea or vomiting episode.
4. Everyone that gets sick with cholera must seek treatment as soon as possible at a medical facility.
5. Dispose of excreta and vomit safely: contain it! If possible, use a latrine to dispose of excreta and vomit. This applies to everyone, including children. If no latrine is available, discreetly wrap it with suitable available materials (e.g. plastic bags, banana leaves) and bury in an isolated area, away from water points and people. Make sure it is well covered.

6. If the outbreak source is positively identified as being food-borne, or becomes food-borne in the course of the outbreak: no raw food please. Boil it, cook it or leave it: avoid undercooked or raw meat, cook all vegetables, clean and cover leftovers, and use clean utensils and dishes (Lamond and Kinjanyui 2012).

## Working with groups to prevent cholera

> Being involved with groups enables individuals to become better organised and mobilised towards collectively addressing their needs.

Working with groups provides an opportunity for the health promoter to help others to develop stronger networks and skills and to find the resources necessary to support their actions. In particular, those groups that can significantly alter relevant health behaviours such as household hygiene through women's groups can make an ideal target population for these types of interventions. Small groups, with sufficient education and capacity building, can also provide a shift to broader issues beyond local concerns, and this can be illustrated through the work of women's groups in Western Samoa (now known as Samoa).

### BOX 7.6: Women's groups in Western Samoa, Polynesia

Women's groups in Western Samoa helped to create a community-centred network for neighbourhood support. The Women's Health Committees (WHC) were prestigious organisations and were supported by the Samoan government through resource allocation, training and regular visits from health workers. The purpose was to develop the skills and competencies of their members in weaning practices and sanitation, which because of diarrhoeal disease had been previously identified as a main cause of infant mortality. The WHC put into force village health regulations relating to sanitation to which all families had to conform. The programme not only brought about improvements in women's health but also their authority, an improved ability to organise and mobilise themselves and to raise funds for other projects. The WHCs became the most influential group in the community and were increasingly involved in addressing a range of local concerns (Thomas 2001).

There is strong evidence that engaging with groups is an effective method for promoting participation and empowering communities with a wide range of benefits such as cost-effectiveness, reductions in mortality and improvements in health (Rosato et al. 2008). However, this is not always a planned feature of large-scale responses. The challenge in disease outbreaks is to use interventions that enable people to move forward from individual concerns to be involved in broader community-managed actions. This gives people a greater capacity and control to work together to take the necessary actions to resolve their needs.

---

**BOX 7.7: Personal protection to address the cholera outbreak in Haiti**

Cholera outbreaks in Haiti are particularly acute during the rainy season. The localised centres of the cholera outbreaks were characterised by areas of poor sanitation, weak health services and the high mobility of people. The Haitian government and its partners implemented a 4-point approach to eliminate cholera in the country, as follows:

1. Rapid response and investigation of all cholera cases led by the Ministry of Health emergency response teams and supported by Untied Nations and non-government organisation partners
2. Increasing community access to clean drinking water and adequate sanitation
3. Strengthening epidemiological surveillance in regard to the number and location of cases and the enhancement of health services at national and local levels
4. The promotion of good hygiene practices via mass media campaigns and group work in community outreach activities

Once a cholera patient had been registered at a treatment centre, his or her home was disinfected and a 'sanitary cordon' was established around the neighbouring 10 houses. Hygiene promotion activities and the provision of cholera kits containing a supply of soap, chlorine tablets to disinfect drinking water and oral rehydration salts were provided to families. Community volunteers called 'brigadiers' had the responsibility of keeping their communities aware, through regular group meetings, of the risk of cholera and how to maintain hygiene practices such as hand-washing and sterilising drinking water (UNICEF 2015b).

---

## POLIOVIRUS OUTBREAKS

Polio (poliomyelitis) is a highly infectious disease caused by a virus. It invades the nervous system and can cause irreversible paralysis in a matter of hours. Polio mainly affects children under 5 years old and is spread through person-to-person contact and through the contamination of water and food. When a child is infected with poliovirus, the virus enters the body through the mouth and multiplies in the intestine. It is then shed into the environment through the faeces where it can spread rapidly through a community, especially in overcrowded conditions of poor hygiene and sanitation. However, if a sufficient number of people, including children, are immunised against polio, the virus is unable to find susceptible people to infect and eventually is eradicated. Most people

---

**BOX 7.8: Herd immunity and the poliovirus**

For polio to occur in a population, there must be an infecting organism, the poliovirus; a susceptible human population; and a cycle of person-to-person transmission. However, if the majority of the population is immune to the poliovirus, the ability of that pathogen to infect another host is reduced, and the cycle of transmission is interrupted. Eventually, the pathogen cannot reproduce and is eradicated. This concept is called herd immunity. However, it is not necessary to vaccinate 100% of the population provided the number of susceptible individuals can be reduced to a sufficiently small number. For example, 80%–86% of individuals in a population must be immune to polio for the susceptible individuals to be protected by herd immunity. When many hosts are vaccinated, especially simultaneously, the transmission of the virus is blocked, and the virus is unable to find another susceptible individual to infect. Because poliovirus can only survive for a short time in the environment (a few weeks at room temperature and a few months at 0°C–8°C), without a human host the virus is eradicated. The oral polio vaccine is 95% effective, and this means that 5 children of every 100 given the vaccine will not develop any immunity and will be susceptible to developing the disease. However, herd immunity provides protection by the immunity of others in the community. If routine immunisation were stopped, the number of unvaccinated, susceptible individuals would however soon exceed the capability of herd immunity to protect them (Global Polio Eradication Initiative 2016).

---

infected with the poliovirus have no signs of illness and are unaware that they have been infected. In others, initial symptoms include fever, fatigue, headache, vomiting, stiffness in the neck and pain in the limbs. The symptomless people can then spread the infection to others before the first case of polio emerges. For this reason, a single confirmed case of polio paralysis is considered to be evidence of an outbreak, particularly in countries where very few cases normally occur.

One in 200 infections of the poliovirus leads to irreversible paralysis, usually in the legs, a condition known as acute flaccid paralysis. All cases of acute flaccid paralysis among children under 15 years of age should be reported. About 40% of people who survive paralytic polio may develop additional symptoms many years after the original illness. This 'post-polio syndrome' includes new progressive muscle weakness. It is not known why only a small percentage of infections lead to paralysis, but reasons may include immune deficiency, pregnancy and physical injury.

## The Global Polio Eradication Initiative

There is no cure for polio, but there are safe and effective vaccines for its prevention, and the eradication strategy is centred on immunising every at-risk child until there is no opportunity for the disease to be transmitted. In 1988 the World Health Assembly adopted a resolution for the worldwide eradication of polio and marked the launch of the Global Polio Eradication Initiative (GPEI). The GPEI achieved a 99% reduction in polio cases worldwide between 1988 and 2000, but this was then followed by a decade of limited eradication (Global Polio Eradication Initiative 2016). The GPEI is a public–private partnership led by national governments and spearheaded by the WHO, Rotary International, the Centers for Disease Control and Prevention and the United Nations Children's Fund. The goal is to eradicate polio worldwide by (1) routine immunisation through oral vaccines, (2) supplementary immunisation, (3) surveillance and (4) targeted mop-up campaigns.

The poliovirus remains endemic in Afghanistan and Pakistan, and the final steps of polio eradication for the GPEI, or what is known as the endgame, are as follows: detect and interrupt all poliovirus transmissions, strengthen immunisation systems, contain the poliovirus and certify interruption of transmission and ensure the remaining investments made to eradicate polio go to the greater cause of improving global health (Global Polio Eradication Initiative 2016).

> Targeting the uptake of vaccination can be an effective approach with large health benefits in some disease outbreaks.

## HEALTH PROMOTION AND THE POLIOVIRUS

The role of health promotion in poliovirus outbreaks is to prevent the transmission of the disease through hygiene promotion campaigns in conjunction with awareness raising about vaccination and the provision of safe water supply and sanitation. Specific behaviours are targeted to prevent the transmission of the disease including hand-washing with soap; safe preparation and storage of food; and importantly, the uptake of vaccination. The health promotion approach uses appropriate channels of communication and community engagement to mobilise communities to play an active role in the containment and eradication of the disease. In Somalia, a rapid response to a poliovirus outbreak between 2013 and 2014 involved 36 polio campaigns which vaccinated 2.3 million children under the age of 5 years over a 2-year period. These efforts successfully resulted in a drop in polio cases from 194 in 2013 to 5 in 2014. The five cases in 2014 had occurred in nomadic-pastoralist families which were difficult to reach due to their remoteness and the ongoing security challenges in the country. The box below explains how these constraints were overcome by using short message service (SMS) – based platforms to help in addressing the polio outbreak.

> The use of commonly available technology such as mobile phones can be an effective channel of communication to raise awareness levels.

> ## BOX 7.9: SMS-based platforms and the poliovirus in Somalia
>
> A health promotion initiative used short message service (SMS) – based platforms to increase awareness about polio in a crisis context in Somalia where mobile phones are used widely; for example, on average 10 people share the benefit of information delivered to one phone even in remote areas. A mobile phone–based technology was introduced as an alternative to house-to-house communication to minimise the security risk to health personnel. The interactive SMS campaign was conducted over a 6-month period including an interactive health education session on polio prevention. The education session focused on community-based behaviours, including hand-washing, how to keep water safe from contamination and vaccination. This component included a 3-day interactive SMS-based session when questions were sent to registered community members and asked to respond to the question. A correct answer prompted them to proceed to the next question. If a question was answered incorrectly, the correct answer would be provided by a text message, and then the participant would be asked to move to the next question. This was designed to reach 100,000 people in 17 districts including in Mogadishu. The campaign also distributed oral rehydration solution, water treatment and soap for hand-washing to participants who had completed the health education sessions. People received a token code (mVoucher) on their phones which could be redeemed at selected prequalified traders for specified resources. Once the code was redeemed, an automatic notification was sent to the system which immediately enrolled the recipient in the second set of education messages. The use of mobile phones was an important aspect of the health promotion approach, especially in areas that were inaccessible and because the infrastructure and technology already existed, this reduced start-up costs. However, consideration was not given to the cost of using SMS to the recipient communities and SMS platforms should always be combined with other channels of communication (Birungi et al. 2016).

## CHALLENGES TO POLIO ERADICATION

An independent evaluation of obstacles to polio eradication has considered the challenges in different countries (World Health Organization 2009). In Afghanistan and Pakistan, the most significant barriers were civil insecurity as well as the movement of large populations between and within countries. The accountability of district health officials was also a problem to adequately monitor the delivery of the vaccination programme. In India, the major challenge was the high transmission of the poliovirus within the population, particularly in Bihar and Uttar Pradesh, which had very poor infrastructures. In Nigeria, the most critical barrier was the low importance given to polio at the local government level, although funding issues, community perceptions of vaccine safety, inadequate social mobilisation and issues with the cold chain also caused challenges. In Angola, Chad and South Sudan, the key barriers were poor health systems and low vaccine coverage. The risk of vaccine-derived polio remains a challenge after the switch to the use of the inactivated vaccine because a small number of people continue to excrete the active virus for years after their initial exposure to the oral vaccine. Other challenges to global polio eradication have been that the oral polio vaccine must be kept at 2°C to 8°C which can be difficult to achieve in hot climates with poor temperature control facilities.

## MIDDLE EAST RESPIRATORY SYNDROME OUTBREAKS

Coronaviruses can cause a range of illnesses in humans, from the common cold to SARS. MERS is a viral respiratory disease caused by a coronavirus (MERS-CoV) that was first identified in Saudi Arabia in 2012. No vaccine or specific treatment is currently available for MERS, and symptoms include fever, cough and shortness of breath. Approximately 36% of reported MERS patients die. The virus seems to cause more severe symptoms in older people, people with weakened immune systems and those with chronic diseases such as cancer and diabetes. The virus does not seem to pass easily from person to person unless there is close contact, such as when providing care to a patient in a healthcare setting, and no sustained community transmission has been documented.

---

### BOX 7.10: Defining cases of MERS-CoV

Public Health England defines a possible case of Middle East respiratory syndrome-coronavirus (MERS-CoV) as any person with severe acute respiratory infection requiring admission to hospital, with symptoms of fever (≥38°C) or history of fever, and cough and with evidence of pulmonary parenchymal disease (e.g. clinical or radiological evidence of pneumonia or acute respiratory distress syndrome not explained by any other infection or aetiology. This is to be accompanied by at least one history of travel to, or residence in, an area where infection with MERS-CoV could have been acquired in the 14 days before symptom onset or close contact during the 14 days before onset of illness with a confirmed case of MERS-CoV infection while the case was symptomatic or a healthcare worker caring for patients with severe acute respiratory infection, regardless of history of travel or use of personal protective equipment or part of a cluster of two or more epidemiologically linked cases within a 2-week period requiring hospital admission, regardless of history of travel. Areas where infection with MERS-CoV could have been acquired include all countries within the geographical Arabian Peninsula, plus countries with cases that cannot be conclusively linked to travel (Public Health England 2016).

Camels are the most likely reservoir host for MERS-CoV in the Middle East and the zoonotic source of infection in humans. A zoonotic disease can be transmitted from animals to people, but more specifically, a zoonotic disease is a disease that normally exists in animals but that can infect humans. The advice given to people is therefore to avoid visiting farms, markets or other places where camels are present and to practice general hygiene measures. These practices include regular hand-washing, before and after touching animals, and avoidance of contact with sick animals. The consumption of raw or undercooked animal products, including camel milk and meat, carries a high risk of infection unless it is pasteurised or cooked.

The epidemiological pattern of MERS-CoV is consistent with sporadic zoonotic cross-infection that can then be amplified within the context of a healthcare setting. Large outbreaks linked to healthcare facilities are a feature of MERS-CoV and are a significant risk factor for infection that is best contained through the rapid implementation of infection prevention and control practices. MERS-CoV in Saudi Arabia occurs throughout the year, with occasional peaks which are a result of large hospital outbreaks and gaps in infection control measures have most likely contributed to these outbreaks. There continues to be a risk of imported cases to other countries such as the Republic of Korea, and health professionals must remain vigilant by using early identification and rapid infection control measures.

The outbreak response to MERS includes conducting risk assessments, developing guidance and training for health authorities on interim surveillance, laboratory testing of cases and infection prevention and control and clinical management. An Emergency Committee under the 2005 International Health Regulations was convened to advise on enhancing surveillance and to review

## BOX 7.11: MERS-CoV in the Republic of Korea

On 29 February 2016, 1644 cases of Middle East respiratory syndrome-coronavirus (MERS-CoV) had been reported to the World Health Organization, with 590 related deaths in Korea. Intensified public health measures including contact tracing, quarantine and isolation of suspected cases and infection prevention and control brought the MERS-CoV under control. The outbreak, which began in May 2015 through the importation of a single case via a traveller from the Middle East, was confined and did not spread outside of healthcare facilities. The response in the Republic of Korea has continued with vigilance for any new cases of MERS-CoV through an early detection system. Healthcare workers are on alert and continue to practice stringent infection prevention and control measures when treating patients to protect themselves, including hand-washing before and after consultation with each patient and wearing a medical mask, eye protection, gown and gloves when treating probable or confirmed MERS-CoV cases (Public Health England 2016).

any unusual patterns of severe acute respiratory infections (SARI) or pneumonia cases. Countries should maintain a high level of vigilance, especially those with large numbers of travellers or migrant workers returning from the Middle East. Surveillance should continue to be enhanced in these countries according to guidelines along with infection prevention and control procedures in healthcare facilities. Confirmed and probable cases of infection with MERS-CoV have to be reported together with information about exposure, testing and treatment to assist with preparedness and response (World Health Organization 2015f).

## HEALTH PROMOTION AND MER-CoV

The role of health promotion to prevent the transmission of MER-CoV is primarily in healthcare settings such as hospitals and clinics to help health workers and patients understand how to protect themselves from the disease. This involves advice on identifying the early symptoms of the disease, using infection prevention and control measures when treating patients, hand-washing before and after consultation with each patient and using personal protective equipment. If a person is confirmed to have, or is being evaluated for, MERS-CoV infection, the prevention procedure is to follow strict prevention steps until medical clearance is given to return to normal activities.

---

### BOX 7.12: The patient-centred clinical method

The patient-centred clinical method applies the principles of empowerment in a professional–patient relationship as follows:

1. The illness and the patient's experience of being ill are explored at the same time.
2. Understanding the person as a whole places the illness into context by considering the following: How does the illness affect the person? How does the person interact with his or her immediate environment? How does the wider environment influence this interaction?
3. The patient and health worker reach a mutual understanding on the nature of the illness its causes and its goals for management, and who is responsible for what.
4. The desirability and applicability to undertake broader health promoting tasks, for example, providing the patient with information or skills about how he or she can wash their hands at home.
5. Gaining a better understanding of the patient–doctor relationship to enhance it, for example, placing a value on the contribution being made by both sides and forming a 'partnership' to address the illness rather than a traditional paternalistic approach.
6. Making a realistic assessment of what can be done to help the patient given constraints in knowledge, time and skill level (Stewart et al. 2003).

The approaches used in health promotion to raise awareness and change behaviour are person-to-person communication, hygiene promotion, educational materials such as leaflets and posters and use of the patient-centred clinical method. Key hygiene messages for preventing MERS-CoV cross-infection are normally developed using rapid assessment techniques as described in Chapter 2. However, the following messages provide an indication of the areas that have been covered in a previous outbreak response using mass media, print materials and face-to-face communication:

1. *Stay home:* You should restrict activities outside your home, except for getting medical care. Do not go to work, school or public areas and do not use public transportation or taxis.
2. *Separate yourself from other people in your home:* As much as possible, you should stay in a different room from other people in your home. Also, you should use a separate bathroom, if available.
3. *Call ahead before visiting your doctor:* Before your medical appointment, call the healthcare provider and tell him or her that you have, or are being, evaluated for MERS-CoV infection. This will help the healthcare provider's office take steps to keep other people from becoming infected.
4. *Wear a facemask:* You should wear a facemask when you are in the same room with other people and when you visit a healthcare provider. If you cannot wear a facemask, the people who live with you should wear one while they are in the same room with you.
5. *Cover your coughs and sneezes:* Cover your mouth and nose with a tissue when you cough or sneeze, or you can cough or sneeze into your sleeve. Throw used tissues in a lined trash can and immediately wash your hands with soap and water.
6. *Wash your hands:* Wash your hands often and thoroughly with soap and water. You can use an alcohol-based hand sanitiser if soap and water are not available and if your hands are not visibly dirty. Avoid touching your eyes, nose and mouth with unwashed hands.
7. *Avoid sharing household items:* You should not share dishes, drinking glasses, cups, eating utensils, towels, bedding or other items with other people in your home. After using these items, you should wash them thoroughly with soap and water.
8. *Monitor your symptoms:* Seek prompt medical attention if your illness is worsening (e.g. difficulty breathing). Before going to your medical appointment, call the healthcare provider and tell him or her that you have, or are being, evaluated for MERS-CoV infection. This will help the healthcare provider's office take steps to keep other people from becoming infected. Ask your healthcare provider to call the local or state health department (Centers for Disease Control and Prevention 2016).

# 8

# Health promotion and vector-borne disease outbreaks

## KEY POINTS

- Community-managed interventions for the self-administration of medicines have proven effective in vector control in difficult to reach areas.
- Health promotion in integrated vector management can identify relevant community perceptions and promote messages that motivate behavioural change.
- Health promotion plays an important role by engaging with communities in mapping and surveillance and by raising awareness about vaccination and personal protection.
- Perceptions change during a disease outbreak, and the response must remain open to new ideas from communities on how to address the problem.
- Health promotion is crucial to mobilise communities to help eradicate vectors that transmit disease such as by reducing localised mosquito-breeding sites.

Vector control is an intervention to reduce or eradicate mammals such as rodents and bats and birds, but mostly insects including mosquitos, ticks, sand flies and fleas that can transmit pathogenic organisms to humans. In particular, it is the mosquito that has the ability to carry and spread disease to humans and cause millions of deaths every year, for example, from malaria, Zika, dengue, chikungunya and yellow fever. Several of the neglected tropical diseases are also transmitted by vectors in Africa, Asia and the Americas, including guinea worm, leishmaniasis, schistosmiasis, onchocerciasis and chagas disease.

The distribution of these diseases is determined by a complex dynamic of environmental and social factors. International travel and trade, agricultural and environmental changes such as unplanned urbanisation have also had an impact on vector-borne diseases.

Vector control programmes are through a modification of environmental, economic and social factors and also include surveillance and reporting systems, training on clinical management, education and the provision of insecticide products and spraying technologies. The role of health promotion is important even with effective treatments because the high associated costs are a barrier to many low-income countries. Community-driven approaches have proven effective in difficult-to-reach areas through the distribution of medicines by using established social networks. Community participation is also important to effectively deliver the measures necessary, such as the use of bed nets, to control vectors. Both vector control and treatment are needed to protect populations against multiple diseases and can be combined to provide an integrated vector management intervention (World Health Organization 2016d).

> Community-managed interventions for the self-administration of medicines have proven effective in vector control in difficult-to-reach areas.

## INTEGRATED VECTOR MANAGEMENT

Integrated vector management (IVM) is a decision-making process that optimises the use of resources for vector control to make it more efficient, cost effective, ecologically sound and sustainable. The IVM approach can address several vectors concurrently because interventions are simultaneously effective against several diseases. The IVM approach uses local evidence, integrates all sectors and engages with households and communities. This is an approach that requires changes in roles and responsibilities and a reorientation of traditional vector-borne disease control programmes within local health systems. Relevant sectors such as agriculture, environment, industry, public works, local government and housing should be incorporated into the IVM strategy to prevent vector proliferation. Planning and implementing IVM involve assessing the epidemiological and vector situation at country level, analysing the local determinants of the disease, identifying and selecting vector control methods, assessing resources and designing locally appropriate implementation strategies. Capacity building, in particular human resource development, can be a challenge, because the IVM strategy requires skilled staff and an adequate infrastructure at both the central and local levels (World Health Organization 2012).

Experiences in South Sudan have shown that strengthened coordination, inter-sectoral collaboration and institutional and technical capacity building for entomological monitoring and evaluation, including the enforcement of appropriate legislation, are crucial to maximise the impact of IVM interventions. An IVM coordinating body with members drawn from ministerial sectors together

> **BOX 8.1: The eradication of onchocerciasis through community-driven initiatives**
>
> Onchocerciasis (river blindness) is a treatable but neglected tropical disease that poses a health risk in endemic areas and is transmitted by the repeated bites of infected blackflies. The goal for the eradication of onchocerciasis is to establish country-led systems in all endemic countries in Africa. After the successful large-scale treatment of populations in affected areas with onchocerciasis, it is possible to stop the transmission of the disease. The eradication of onchocerciasis in Africa has used a community-driven process that enables treatment in difficult-to-reach remote and conflict-affected areas through the distribution of medicines by using established social networks. In addition, trained community volunteers help to reinforce the traditional healthcare system. In the rural populations of sub-Saharan Africa where health systems are weak and under-resourced, the community-driven strategy is proving to be a successful approach in reducing the disease at low cost. Community-driven treatment with ivermectin promotes active participation and local ownership. Communities collectively plan their own distribution systems, decide who distributes the medicine and decide where and when it is delivered. Communities take charge and the role of ministries of health and non-government organisations is to support them in achieving their goals (Amazigo 2008).

with establishing a vector control unit within the Ministry of Health were also identified as an important aspect of the national programme (Chanda et al. 2013).

> Health promotion in integrated vector management can identify relevant community perceptions and promote messages that motivate behavioural change.

In this chapter, I address the role of health promotion in the prevention of vector-borne disease outbreaks through examples from the recent Zika virus response, the new threat from a mammalian source of Nipah disease, chikungunya disease and the re-emergent threat of yellow fever.

## ZIKA VIRUS OUTBREAKS

The Zika virus is transmitted through an infected mosquito, primarily *Aedes aegypti*, but can also be transmitted through sexual intercourse and is usually confirmed through laboratory tests on blood. People infected with the Zika virus have symptoms that include a mild fever, skin rash, conjunctivitis, muscle and joint pain, malaise and headache. These symptoms normally last for 2–7 days. In 2015, Brazil reported an association between Zika virus infection and Guillain–Barré syndrome, a rapid-onset muscle weakness in adults caused by the immune system damaging the peripheral nervous system; and microcephaly, a medical condition in newborn babies in which the brain does not develop properly, resulting in a smaller than normal head (World Health Organization 2016a).

## HEALTH PROMOTION AND THE ZIKA VIRUS

Vector control and personal protection are the key measures to prevent Zika virus infection. Personal protection can include wearing clothes that cover as much of the body as possible, using physical barriers such as window and door screens, sleeping under mosquito nets and using insect repellents to protect from mosquito bites. It also includes the use of condoms for safer sexual intercourse. Health promotion has a role to play through awareness-raising campaigns and engaging with communities to help reduce the localised breeding sites of mosquitoes and peer education to promote the use of condoms. Vector control

### BOX 8.2: Zika control and pregnancy in Puerto Rico

In Puerto Rico, feedback was gained from pregnant women about vector control activities being considered for the Zika virus. It was important to determine whether pregnant women would accept or reject each activity and to determine their opinions about the acceptability of behaviour change. Twelve messages were developed for pregnant women using plain language and line drawings to illustrate the text. The messages covered vector control activities in regard to removing standing water, protective clothing, repellent use, bed nets, different types of residual spray, participation in community clean-up campaigns and condom use. The methodology used three focus group discussions with 8–10 pregnant women in which the key messages and images were shown, read aloud and discussed. The focus group discussions were followed up with 27 in-depth Interviews. The participants were asked about their Zika knowledge and trusted information sources and given the opportunity to offer reactions to messages depicting protective behaviours. The pregnant women interviewed did not reject or oppose any of the messages or behaviours, but they expressed feelings of anxiety and vulnerability in regard to the Zika virus and microcephaly. The pregnant women supported neighbourhood, community and government action in regard to vector control. They preferred actions that were familiar and under their control such as protective clothing and bed nets rather than actions that were unfamiliar such as aerial spraying. The findings of the assessment were built into the Puerto Rico communication plan to help to revise messages, text and illustrations for health promotion materials (Prue 2016).

can be supported by local health authorities through, for example, widespread spraying of insecticides.

In South America in 2015, the Zika outbreak response was modified to reduce the risk of transmission from sexual intercourse and in resulting pregnancy complications. The communication messaging was adjusted to include advice on safer sex by using a condom or abstaining from sexual activity, especially for the partners of pregnant women living in or returning from areas affected by the Zika virus. In addition, people returning from areas where local transmission of the Zika virus occurred were requested to adopt safer sexual practices or abstain from sex for at least 8 weeks after their return, even if they did not have symptoms. Men with Zika virus symptoms were given the advice to adopt safer sexual practices or consider abstinence for at least 6 months. The messaging also advised those people planning a pregnancy to wait at least 8 weeks before trying to conceive if no symptoms of Zika virus infection appeared, or 6 months if one or both members of the couple were symptomatic (World Health Organization 2016a).

## THE ZIKA STRATEGIC RESPONSE FRAMEWORK AND HEALTH PROMOTION

The World Health Organization's 'Zika Strategic Response Framework' focusses on communicating risks with women of child-bearing age, pregnant women, their partners, households and communities, so that people have the information they need to protect themselves. Other aspects include IVM, sexual and reproductive health counselling and health education. The framework outlines four main approaches to support national governments and communities in preventing and managing the Zika virus: detection, prevention, care and support and research (World Health Organization 2016a). The role of health promotion in each approach is described below.

### Detection

It is important to develop, strengthen and implement integrated surveillance systems at all levels to provide accurate epidemiological and entomological information to guide the response. The role of health promotion in detection is in engaging communities in activities such as mapping mosquito breeding sites and helping authorities in undertaking surveillance. An example is surveillance and early reporting of Guillain–Barré syndrome. Raising public awareness about the importance of early reporting of symptoms and suspected Zika cases is also a key health promotion activity using both traditional and mass media approaches such as local radio, posters and person-to-person communication.

Health promotion plays an important role by engaging with communities in mapping and surveillance and by raising awareness about vaccination and personal protection.

## Prevention

Risk communication and community engagement are key to preventing the spread of the Zika virus in conjunction with vector management and changing sexual practices. Controlling the spread of the virus requires a multi-faceted approach, which is not only concerned with vector control but also with protecting individuals, especially pregnant women and women of reproductive age, and preventing unwanted pregnancies through supporting access to sexual and reproductive health services. This includes the following:

- Implementing IVM to efficiently use resources
- Targeting all life stages of the *Aedes* mosquito: egg, larva, pupa and adult
- Reducing the risk of sexual transmission and other possible routes of transmission
- Coordinating, collaborating and partnering with stakeholders from government (e.g. municipalities, ministries of education, health, social services, water and sanitation, etc.) and civil society (non-government organisations, private sector, faith-based associations, churches)
- Engaging and empowering communities in mosquito control and prevention behaviours at the environmental, household, school, business and personal levels
- Developing relevant risk communication and behaviour change strategies and materials

Communication messaging for protection against the Zika virus are also key health promotion activities. Key messages are normally developed using rapid assessment techniques as described in Chapter 2. However, messaging for

---

**BOX 8.3: Farmer field schools**

Farmer field schools give practical, field-based education during weekly meetings to help farmers acquire skills to analyse their ecosystem and to make informed decisions on how to grow healthy crops with less use of pesticides. Communication skills and a strengthening of farmers' groups are important aspects of the training. Integrated pest management programmes contribute to disease control by reducing the use of pesticides and thereby the risk for the development of resistance in disease vectors. In one pilot project in rice ecosystems in Sri Lanka, mosquito vector control activities in agricultural and home environments were carried out while also increasing rice productivity. A 60% increase in the use of bed nets was also recorded, indicating an increased awareness about personal protection against mosquitoes (World Health Organization 2006a).

preventing the transmission of the Zika virus can usually be organised around the following seven pillars:

1. Community actions to control the day-biting *Aedes* vector (such as eliminating breeding sites) and personal protective actions to prevent the bite of this mosquito
2. Age-appropriate and culturally acceptable health education for anyone who may be sexually active, accompanied by counselling and health services as appropriate
3. Risk communication for healthcare workers, who need the knowledge, tools and skills to effectively and empathetically counsel, advise and offer appropriate services
4. National and local risk communication and community engagement plans with all relevant stakeholders for effective and proactive action against this threat
5. Information and education so that travellers and their sexual partners know and understand the risks, and also to prevent unnecessary negative decisions for travel and trade
6. Operational research to understand knowledge, attitudes and practices and so inform ongoing interventions
7. Coordination among key responders, such as affected governments, United Nations, non-government organisations and other international agencies; national and local actors; researchers; and social science networks

## Care and support

Strengthening health and social systems at the national and community levels to provide appropriate services and to support individuals, families, and communities is essential in a Zika outbreak. This primarily focusses on the needs of women and girls of childbearing age and children born with complications from the infection, families, communities at risk and people with Guillain–Barré syndrome. Strengthening health and social systems includes the following: identifying and treating people with Zika virus infection complications, regardless of gender and disability; addressing the psychological and economic impact of the complications, in part by providing adequate psychosocial and mental health support; dealing with the long-term implications of children affected by microcephaly and other complications; addressing non-medical consequences of the virus such as stigma, reduced income and increased poverty; giving pregnant women access to point-of-care technology for detecting Zika virus infection and, if such is the case, access to counselling and psychosocial advice, and, if possible, to ultrasonography to monitor foetal growth; and developing capacities to recognise and care for patients with severe Guillain–Barré syndrome.

The role of health promotion is to provide accurate information about access to sexual and reproductive healthcare and services for all women and adolescent girls of reproductive age in the affected areas. This includes access to family planning, counselling, contraceptive services, safe abortion services and post-abortion care. Ensuring all groups are included in national response plans and related Zika prevention activities are also carried out as a part of health promotion in coordination with local authorities and non-government partners. Health and social systems need to adjust to a greater demand from families affected by the complications of the Zika virus for rehabilitative services, social assistance and protection, psychosocial support and specialised healthcare and education. Multiple disciplines will be required to ensure the effective delivery of essential health services and the management of Zika complications, delivered by a skilled health and social care workforce.

> Perceptions change during a disease outbreak and the response must remain open to new ideas from communities on how to address the problem.

## Research

Systematic research that tracks the perception of risk and the uptake of protective behaviours will enable the development of effective communication and community engagement approaches. Evidence is also needed to strengthen public involvement to prevent, detect and control the Zika virus and to self-manage its complications (World Health Organization 2016a).

## NIPAH VIRUS INFECTION OUTBREAKS

The Nipah virus (NiV) is an emerging zoonotic disease with the potential to cause a disease outbreak as there is currently no cure or vaccine to treat humans. The UK Wellcome Trust, a founding member of the Coalition for Epidemic Preparedness Innovations, has identified the Nipah virus, Lassa fever and Middle East respiratory syndrome as likely causes of a future global health emergency and have been prioritised for the research and development of diagnostic tests, vaccines and treatments (Muzundar 2017).

The NiV infection is a *Henipavirus*, a genus of RNA viruses naturally harboured by pteropid fruit bats (flying foxes) and several species of microbats. The finding of henipaviruses in Africa, Australia and Asia indicates that it has the potential to become endemic in a country (Drexler et al. 2009). The term 'Nipah' refers to the place, Kampung Baru Sungai Nipah in Negeri Sembilan state, Malaysia, the source of the human case from which the virus was first isolated. Nipah virus was first identified in April 1999, when it caused an outbreak of neurological and respiratory disease on pig farms in Malaysia, resulting in 257 human cases, including 105 human deaths and the culling of 1 million pigs. Symptoms of infection during the outbreak were primarily encephalitic in humans, and it was initially diagnosed as Japanese encephalitis. The Ministry of Health launched a nationwide campaign to educate people on the dangers

> ## BOX 8.4: Preventing Nipah virus infection in Bangladesh
>
> Eight outbreaks of the Nipah virus (NiV) infection were reported in Bangladesh between 2001 and 2009. Bangladesh is densely populated, and date palm sap harvesting is a common profession. A primary pathway of transmission from bats to people in Bangladesh was through the contamination of raw date sap as bats also feed on the date palm. The first preventive measure was therefore in limiting exposure of villagers to NiV-contaminated fresh date palm sap; however, date palm sap collection provides critical income to low-income collectors and is a seasonal national delicacy enjoyed by millions of people every year. Steps to make date palm sap consumption safer include diverting more of the production to molasses where the sap is cooked at temperatures above the level that NiV can survive and limiting bat access to date palm trees where the sap will be consumed fresh (Luby et al. 2009).

of Japanese encephalitis and its vector, *Culex* mosquitoes. However, it was later noticed that people who had been vaccinated against Japanese encephalitis were not protected. Because the disease can be difficult to diagnose based on clinical signs alone, surveillance tools are essential for the NiV and include reliable laboratory assays for early detection of the disease in people and livestock. The transmission of the NiV from flying foxes to pigs was thought to be due to an overlap between bat habitats and piggeries in Malaysia. Eight more outbreaks of the NiV have occurred since 1999, all within Bangladesh, Singapore and neighbouring parts of India (Lo Presti et al. 2015).

In humans, NiV typically presents as fever, headache, drowsiness, abdominal pain, vomiting, problems with swallowing and blurred vision. About one-quarter of the patients have seizures and about 60% become comatose and might need mechanical ventilation.

## HEALTH PROMOTION AND NIPAH VIRUS INFECTION

In the absence of a vaccine, raising awareness of the risk factors and educating people about measures that can reduce exposure to the NiV are the most common preventive measures to reduce infection.

## Animal-to-human transmission

To reduce the risk of animal-to-human NiV transmission, information is provided about the use of protective equipment such as gloves, gowns, eyewear and boots when handling sick animals, meat and during slaughtering. Good hand hygiene should be practised at all times, especially before leaving farms and abattoirs.

Specific control measures to reduce the risk of animal-to-human NiV transmission focus on the following:

- Avoiding contact with fruit bats and infected animals
- Ensuring that fruit bats are not able to roost close to animal pens
- Reducing bats' access to foodstuffs that can act as a means of transmission such as date palm sap
- Testing possible bat source for the presence of NiV or serological evidence of infection
- Using appropriate protective equipment
- Slaughtering infected pigs and burying or incinerating the carcasses
- Restricting the movement of pigs from infected farms or designated areas

Other important control measures have been a ban on pig production in the regions affected, biosecurity practices and decreasing the likelihood of the bat reservoir coming into contact with pig production. Control measures can include eradication by mass culling of infected and in-contact animals After culling, the burial sites are disinfected as well as the contaminated areas and equipment.

## Human-to-human transmission

To reduce the risk of human-to-human transmission, information is provided about the avoidance of unnecessary close physical contact with infected people including isolation, along with standard, droplet and contact precautions. Asymptomatic contacts require further education on transmission prevention and on the early signs and symptoms of illness. In healthcare settings or where there is a risk of exposure of caregivers, the role of health promotion is to prevent the transmission of the NiV by helping both carers and patients to understand how to protect themselves. This involves advice on identifying the early symptoms of the disease, using infection prevention and control measures when treating patients, hand-washing before and after consultation with each patient and using personal protective equipment. The approaches used in health promotion to raise awareness and change behaviour are person-to-person communication and hygiene promotion supplemented with the use of educational materials such as leaflets and flashcards.

## CHIKUNGUNYA DISEASE OUTBREAKS

Chikungunya disease has been identified in more than 60 countries in Asia, Africa, Europe and the Americas. Infections of chikungunya in Africa were at relatively low levels for many years, but between 1999 and 2000 there was a large outbreak in the Democratic Republic of the Congo and in 2007 there was another outbreak in Gabon. A large outbreak of chikungunya in India occurred between 2006 and 2007 and in Indonesia, the Maldives, Myanmar and Thailand there were more than 1.9 million reported cases between 2005 and 2016. In 2007, the disease was reported for the first time in Europe, in a localised outbreak in northeastern Italy. There were 197 cases recorded during this outbreak, and it confirmed that mosquito-borne outbreaks by *Aedes albopictus* are possible in Europe (World Health Organization 2016b).

The chikungunya virus is transmitted by a mosquito vector, most commonly *Ae. aegypti* and *Ae. albopictus*. These mosquitoes are active throughout daylight hours with peaks of activity in the early morning and late afternoon, both inside and outside buildings. *Aedes aegypti* is confined within the tropics and subtropics. *Aedes albopictus* occurs in temperate and colder regions and breeds in a wide range of localised sites such as bamboo stumps and vehicle tyres. This diversity of habitats explains the abundance of *Ae. albopictus* in rural as well as peri-urban areas. *Aedes aegypti* is more closely associated with human habitation and can use indoor breeding sites including water storage containers (World Health Organization 2016b).

Chikungunya is characterised by an abrupt onset of fever frequently accompanied by joint and muscle pain, headache, nausea, fatigue and a rash. The symptoms can last for a few days and most patients recover fully, but symptoms can persist for several months or even years. Occasional cases of eye, neurological and heart complications have been reported, as well as gastrointestinal complaints. Serious complications are not common, but in older people the disease can be the cause of death. Symptoms that are mild may go unrecognised or be misdiagnosed in areas where dengue occurs. There is no cure for chikungunya and prevention focusses on vector control and personal protection.

## HEALTH PROMOTION AND CHIKUNGUNYA OUTBREAKS

The general response to a chikungunya outbreak involves the preparation of management plans, improving reporting systems, training on clinical management, disease diagnosis and vector control. The health promotion response to a chikungunya outbreak focusses on health messaging and community engagement activities for vector control and prevention such as advice regarding personal protection, for example:

- The proximity of mosquito vector breeding sites to human habitation is a significant risk factor for chikungunya. Prevention and control relies heavily on reducing the number of natural and artificial water-filled habitats that support the breeding of the mosquitoes. This depends on the ability to mobilise communities and on the use of insecticides to kill mosquitoes, applied to surfaces in and around breeding sites and in containers to kill the immature larvae.
- For personal protection against chikungunya, clothing which minimises skin exposure is used as well as repellents. Insecticide-treated mosquito nets afford good protection for sleeping during the daytime or for people confined to bed. Other precautions include window screens and door curtains to prevent mosquitoes from entering dwellings (World Health Organization 2016b).

> ## BOX 8.5: Public perceptions of the *Aedes aegypti* mosquito in Brazil
>
> One study in Brazil explored how communication about the *Aedes aegypti* mosquito could be turned into preventive actions by better understanding the perceptions of different actors regarding the proliferation of the vector. The study undertook 10 focus groups conducted in March 2016 with a variety of stakeholders including municipal managers, health agencies, local leaders and members of the public. The public perception was that there is little risk of long-term symptoms with dengue and for the Zika disease the serious issues were only for pregnant women. Chikungunya had serious symptoms for everyone including severe pain in the body for prolonged periods which can greatly influence function and quality of life. People were found to have a good knowledge about controlling the proliferation of the *Ae. aegypti* mosquito, but there were not sufficiently convincing arguments about why it was important to actually prevent transmission. People were aware of ways to protect themselves individually such as using long-sleeved shirts, mosquito repellent and bed nets. However, few people followed this advice because of the hot climate and the high price of repellents. Health promoters reported that they were overburdened and did not have the necessary materials or training to carry out educational actions regarding the *Ae. aegypti* mosquito (PLAN 2016).

## YELLOW FEVER OUTBREAKS

Yellow fever is an acute viral haemorrhagic disease transmitted by infected mosquitoes belonging to the *Aedes* and *Haemogogus* genera and that live in different habitats; some breed around houses (domestic), others in the jungle (wild) and some in both habitats (semi-domestic). The symptoms of yellow fever include headache, jaundice, muscle pain, fever, nausea, vomiting and fatigue. A small proportion of patients who contract the virus develop severe symptoms, and approximately one-half of those die within 7 to 10 days. Yellow fever is difficult to diagnose, especially during its early stages, and can be confused with malaria, leptospirosis, viral hepatitis and other haemorrhagic fevers such as dengue. The virus remains endemic in 47 countries in Africa and 13 in Central and South America. Outbreaks of yellow fever occur when infected people introduce the virus into heavily populated areas with a high vector density and where most people have no access to vaccination. In these conditions, infected mosquitoes can quickly transmit the yellow fever virus throughout the whole population (World Health Organization 2016e).

> Vaccination is the most important means of preventing several disease outbreaks including yellow fever, polio and cholera. Health promotion can effectively promote the use of vaccination services and raise awareness about the risks of infection.

Vaccination is the most important means of preventing yellow fever. In high-risk areas where coverage is low, prompt recognition and control of an outbreak are achieved by using mass vaccination. Under-reporting can be a problem; therefore, just one laboratory-confirmed case of yellow fever in an unvaccinated population is considered an outbreak and must be fully investigated. Investigation teams must assess and respond to the outbreak with both health emergency measures and longer term immunisation plans (World Health Organization 2016f).

---

### BOX 8.6: Yellow fever control in the Côte d'Ivoire

In September 2001, yellow fever cases were confirmed in 5 of the 10 communes in Abidjan in the Côte d'Ivoire. Urban yellow fever can spread rapidly among a dense population such as the 3.5 million people living in Abidjan. An operations centre was established to coordinate activities in epidemiology, the immunisation campaign and vector control. Vaccines and safe injection equipment were provided through an International Coordinating Group for Emergency Vaccine Provision. Vaccines were provided. The mass campaign immunised 2.9 million people over only a 10-day period (World Health Organization 2015d).

---

Several vaccination strategies are used to protect against yellow fever outbreaks including the following: routine infant immunisation, mass vaccination campaigns designed to increase coverage in countries at risk, and the vaccination of travellers going to yellow fever endemic areas. In accordance with the International Health Regulations (see Chapter 1), countries have the right to require travellers to provide a certificate of yellow fever vaccination.

The World Health Organization is the Secretariat for the International Coordinating Group (ICG) for Yellow Fever Vaccine Provision. The ICG maintains an emergency stockpile of yellow fever vaccines to ensure rapid response to outbreaks in high-risk countries. In 2006, the yellow fever initiative was launched to secure a global vaccine supply and boost population immunity through

---

### BOX 8.7: Yellow fever in the Democratic Republic of the Congo

In August 2016 amid the potential of a yellow fever outbreak in the Democratic Republic of the Congo, the World Health Organization initiated a mass vaccine campaign assisted by key partners such 'Doctors Without Borders'. Global supplies of the vaccine were limited and had not fully stockpiled; therefore, the World Health Organization decided to approve a lower dose, issuing inoculations of one-fifth of the normal dose. This provided protection for 1 year, rather than for a lifetime. However, by September 2016 more than 7 million people had been vaccinated against yellow fever in the Kinshasa province (The Guardian 2016).

vaccination. The initiative, led by the World Health Organization, supported by United Nations Children's Fund and by national governments, has a particular focus on high endemic countries in Africa where the disease is most prominent. More than 105 million people have been vaccinated and no yellow fever outbreaks were reported in 2015 (World Health Organization 2015d).

## HEALTH PROMOTION AND YELLOW FEVER OUTBREAKS

The role of health promotion in yellow fever outbreaks is to increase the uptake of vaccination through public awareness campaigns and to help reduce the number of mosquitoes through social mobilisation by destroying the breeding sites of the developing larvae, as well as the following:

- Reducing the number of natural and artificial water-filled habitats that support the breeding of the mosquitoes. This depends on the ability to mobilise communities and on the use of insecticides to kill mosquitoes, applied to surfaces in and around breeding sites and in containers to kill the immature larvae.
- Personal protection clothing which minimises skin exposure is used as well as repellents. Insecticide-treated mosquito nets afford good protection for sleeping during the daytime or for people confined to bed. Other precautions include window screens and door curtains to prevent mosquitoes from entering dwellings.

> Health promotion is crucial to mobilise communities to help eradicate vectors that transmit disease such as by reducing localised mosquito breeding sites.

Key messages for yellow fever outbreaks are normally developed using rapid assessment techniques as described in Chapter 2. However, below is a guide for developing messages that can be used after proper adaptation to the local culture and language and for producing health promotion materials before and during the campaign and then after the outbreak has finished.

## Health promotion messages and yellow fever

| Key messages | Proposed health promotion activities |
|---|---|
| **Implement before and during the campaign** | |
| Every single person in the community needs a yellow fever vaccine. | Media messaging including TV and popular radio stations broadcasted in local languages. |
| The yellow fever vaccine is safe and protects you for life (if a full dose is given). | Identify a role model (being vaccinated or talking about vaccination) for the spots, TV, |

*Continued*

| Key messages | Proposed health promotion activities |
|---|---|
| | posters, and other communication materials for mass distribution. Place posters in vaccination/health centres. |
| Just be vaccinated and continue to your daily routine, no need to change anything. Vaccine is safe and real/true. | Production and placement of posters and street banners with key messages placed in busy markets, streets, churches, schools and taxi and bus stops. Advocate with schools: have teachers provide key messages to students; develop student brigades (older kids) to promote key messages with their neighbours. Advocate with religious leaders, community leaders and business leaders so they communicate key messages to their followers. Social mobilisation: identify community leaders to communicate key messages in their community. Recruit and train social mobilisers to work door to door in priority communities. Identify 'champions' to advocate for vaccination. |

**Implement after campaign or if no vaccination programme**

| | |
|---|---|
| Mosquitoes transmit yellow fever when they bite. Mosquitoes breed in standing water and bite during the day. Get rid of standing water in your house and outside your house. | Constant media key messaging including TV and popular radio stations. Production and placement of posters and street banners with key messages placed in busy markets, streets, churches and schools. Advocate with schools: have teachers provide key messages to students. Advocate with religious leaders, community leaders and business leaders so they communicate key messages to their followers. |

*Continued*

| Key messages | Proposed health promotion activities |
|---|---|
| **Implement after the outbreak** | |
| Every single person in the community needs a yellow fever vaccine for life-long protection. | Media key messaging including TV and popular radio stations. |
| Bring all children to health centre for routine vaccination. | Production and placement of posters with messages placed in clinics, busy markets, streets, churches and schools. |
| Get rid of standing water in your house and outside your house to get rid of mosquitoes. | Advocate with schools: have teachers provide messages to students. |
| Mosquitoes transmit yellow fever when they bite. | Advocate with religious leaders, community leaders and business leaders so they can communicate key messages to their followers. |

Adapted from http://wwwnc.cdc.gov/travel/diseases/yellow-fever. Accessed 14 October 2016.

## HEALTH PROMOTION AND VACCINATION CAMPAIGNS

Vaccination is the most important means of preventing many diseases and with prompt recognition it can and control an outbreak in conjunction with health promotion interventions. The role of health promotion is to raise public awareness about the availability of vaccination with communication strategies, for example, hygiene promotion campaigns and the provision of safe water supply and sanitation. Health promotion can also mobilise communities to play an active role in the containment and eradication of a disease at a localised level, for example, by destroying the breeding sites of mosquitoes and more effectively with the spraying of insecticides and the use of insecticide-treated bed nets.

In particular, the role of health promotion in the delivery of a vaccination campaign can be improved by ensuring that the following key activities are addressed: building small-scale activities, advocacy activities, communication and social mobilisation and operational steps. Operational steps involve the following: identifying the district communications focal point; developing a local communication action plan; defining the main messages; getting the right media mix, including the use of banners and posters; training communicators and mobilisers; and working with networks (World Health Organization 2015d).

### The key activities

#### BUILDING SMALL-SCALE ACTIVITIES

A health campaign covers the whole country or a set of regions; however, the district health centre is the focal point for health workers to prepare before the campaign starts. In a mass vaccination campaign, communication and community engagement take place primarily at the district level, usually through the district health centre. To gain support, the vaccination team must engage, as appropriate, with local chiefs, the traditional authorities and the district managers to ensure that these key partners are committed to the campaign. Not only does their participation provide a positive example but also they are able to provide or advise on important activities such as reaching marginalised groups or isolated families.

## ADVOCACY ACTIVITIES

Advocacy activities influence decision makers through a variety of channels, including meetings between various levels of government and civil society organisations at the community level, on the need for local action. Media advocacy highlights the relevance of the campaign, puts issues on the public agenda and encourages local media to cover related topics regularly and in a responsible manner to raise awareness of possible solutions and ongoing problems. District and provincial level managers should have a mechanism to regularly share information, for example, by jointly attending briefings.

## COMMUNICATION AND SOCIAL MOBILISATION

Communication aims to change knowledge, attitudes and practices among key stakeholders. The formative research should explore the reasons why people do or do not take action on the information they receive and the messages adapted accordingly and then focus on changing the actual behaviour by addressing the causes identified. Communication methods include mass media channels, such as radio, posters, banners, flyers and mobile phones. Social mobilisation brings together community members and other stakeholders to strengthen participation to generate a dialogue, negotiation and a consensus about action.

# The operational steps

## IDENTIFYING THE DISTRICT COMMUNICATION FOCAL POINT

Each sub-regional area should have a communication focal point. This is a key person in the campaign for implementation and the coordination of activities at the provincial and district levels. Other ongoing campaigns might include polio, measles and the distribution of mosquito nets; therefore, it is necessary to support this position to ensure better coordination between the different activities.

## DEVELOPING A LOCAL ACTION PLAN

A local assessment by the focal point is conducted by using information to establish the success of the campaign in a specific district. Local communication action plans must have the following components: the number of activities; tasks for each activity; target group or audience for each activity; responsible person, organisation or partnership for each activity; outcome of each activity; and timelines for each activity.

## DEFINING THE MAIN MESSAGES

The main messages in the campaign must capture the necessary details to communicate these to the population, often by mobilisers when they visit schools, public places or homes. Journalists need to know what yellow fever is, why the campaign is taking place and how the vaccines will be administered. Decision makers, politicians and religious leaders need to understand the logistics of the campaign and why they are involved in the implementation.

## GETTING THE RIGHT MEDIA MIX

Getting the right media mix and messages is the basis for a good communication strategy and is discussed in Chapter 3. The use of the right media and message mix is dependent on the sociocultural context of the disease outbreak; therefore, what works in one context may not be effective in another. Health promotion includes a broad range of ideas and concepts, many of which have not been fully tested in practice. A major challenge is how to apply the correct theory (the science) to the appropriate practice context (the art). Achieving both the 'art and science' of health promotion is possible through the selection of the best strategy for a particular programme and sociocultural context.

## TRAINING COMMUNICATORS AND MOBILISERS

For focal points and mobilisers, the most effective training should include the following components: objectives of the campaign; target group(s); main messages; criteria for recruiting mobilisers; functions of the mobilisers before, during and after the campaign; and samples of the visual materials.

Recruiting communicators and mobilisers is an important step that requires candidates in the locality who are credible and capable of completing the work. Before the campaign, the day-to-day activities of the mobilisers will include talking to village members; identifying key partners; conducting meetings; preparing communication materials such as posters, brochures and banners; and advertising the campaign in public places. During the campaign, they will promote the participation of organised community groups and other community members such as teachers, parents and children.

---

### BOX 8.8: Getting the right media and message mix in vaccination campaigns

For vaccination campaigns in Sierra Leone, Guinea, Côte d'Ivoire and the Central African Republic, the most efficient channels of communication were a combination of the town crier + radio + short message service. However, banners and posters were also used in the health centres where vaccination posts are located and in schools, mosques, churches, markets, shops and other public places as informational tools to spread messages about the vaccination campaign at a localised level (World Health Organization 2015d).

## WORKING WITH NETWORKS

Social networks are considered a key communication channel in many countries, and an investment for their establishment and maintenance allows a better interaction between its members. Social networks offer people the opportunity to strengthen their relationships; spread positive health behaviours; and build their knowledge, skills and ability to cope in a stressful situation such as a disease outbreak.

# 9

# Addressing rumour, resistance and security issues

---

> **KEY POINTS**
>
> - Trust is difficult to maintain when local people receive information that does not match with their own experiences.
> - Conflict can be resolved in our everyday work by being good listeners and inviting people to simply clarify any issues of concern.
> - Clear statements of military activities in the disease outbreak can help to alleviate community concerns.
> - Community-led quarantines are important in the success of outbreak responses.
> - Community management of cross-border movement includes activities that are crucial to a successful response such as community policing and contact tracing.

Non-compliant behaviour is part of a cycle of unwillingness to change traditional practices that can be made worse by experiences of poor service delivery and weak information flow. This can become heightened in an atmosphere of fear and resistance and was a key issue in Guinea, Liberia and Sierra Leone during the Ebola virus disease outbreak. However, the nature of the resistance changed as the outbreak developed, and although the total number of non-compliant incidents decreased, the level of violence increased and was confined to specific localities (Laverack and Manoncourt 2015). The violent incidents were geographically mapped, forewarning agencies and providing a better understanding of the causes of the resistance. In Guinea, for example, some communities had a history of conflict that was linked to oppressive political action. The causes of resistance were a combination of rumour, misinformation and poor professional practice. Systematic efforts to collect and analyse rumours were initiated in Liberia, and it was found that misinformation continued even towards the end of the response, for example, in regard to decommissioning and back-to-school activities (Internews 2015).

> Trust is difficult to maintain when local people receive information that does not match with their own experiences.

Building trust can be time-consuming and requires skilled community workers that are familiar with the diversity of cultures present in the population (Dhillon and Kelly 2015). However, systematic community engagement techniques (see Chapter 5) can be used to 'fast-track' this process without affecting the integrity of the response. The advice given, as requested by communities, should be practical and about the risk factors of transmission, and how to reduce risks when caring for the sick, as well as provide resources to help to put this advice into practice (Chandler et al. 2014).

## COMMUNITY RUMOURS

A rumour, in the context of a disease outbreak, can be defined as an unverified but relevant statement of information spread among people (DiFonzo and Bordia 2007). Gaps in knowledge, poor delivery of communication approaches, strong traditional beliefs and negative experiences of health service delivery can all contribute to the creation of rumours. Health facilities, for example, can be a source of disease transmission and some patients that are admitted later die. This can reinforce community perceptions of poor practice and can lead to rumours of professional abuse. Rumours can be linked to issues of structural violence that have contributed to the spread of a disease such as the unfair distribution of resources, vaccination coverage or the provision of health and education facilities. Structural violence refers to the way institutions inflict avoidable harm on people's lives and health, often embedded into society. It is not caused by any single institution but is a combination of overlapping policies and practices that produce interrelated inequalities. Structural violence is also often historical and part of a legacy of the distrust of government caused by a failure to provide basic services and public security (Wilkinson and Leach 2014). For example, a rumour that embodies the experience of structural violence is 'the government is injecting people with Ebola to increase the number of cases to get more money from the international community' (Reuters 2014). Rumours can also play an important role as a means for people to come to terms with the consequences of a disease outbreak in relation to problematic political, economic and social experiences. In fact, if rumours disappear, people can act as if the disease outbreak had never existed. Consequently, behaviours to prevent the transmission of the disease such as safe burials are not adhered to and this can make the transmission even more likely to happen (Wigmore 2016).

Rumours can be spread through a variety of channels including social media, mass media and person-to-person contact. Examples of rumours that occurred during the Ebola virus disease outbreak in West Africa include the following: 'Vaccinators are here to give you Ebola'; 'Government workers intentionally infect people with Ebola to continue receiving money from the donors';

> **BOX 9.1: Witch planes and Ebola in Sierra Leone**
>
> In Sierra Leone, witch planes are believed to be tiny aeroplanes that are used to transport witches from one place to another; for example, a groundnut shell or animals can be used as witch planes. Occasionally, in this magic world there are accidents in which a witch plane could crash and bring a sickness. A witch plane crash in Port Loko, Sierra Leone, related to a conflict between two chiefs after an election, was believed by local people to have brought Ebola (Wigmore 2016).

'thermometers are instruments to infect people intentionally'; and 'government workers – health and school teachers – are being paid to spread Ebola' (Ministry of Health 2015).

Rumours can directly influence an outbreak response; for example, in Pakistan in 2011 a rumour was started that the US government was using immunisation campaigns to sterilise the local population. Pakistan reported the world's highest number of polio cases in 2011; and even with the support of political leaders, polio workers were kidnapped, beaten and killed in remote areas of the country (Warraich 2009). Rumour can often have an element of logic, but this logic can adversely affect compliance. In Wellington, Freetown, for example, a rumour suggested that sachets found in rice rations provided by the response (probably a desiccant used to keep the rice fresh and marked 'poison') were sachets intended to contaminate the food. This caused people to resist or to violate quarantine measures (Wigmore 2016). Rumours also have a causal effect on attitudes and behaviours such as the denial of an illness being attributed to a disease or the hiding of sick people and dead bodies. This is a cycle of rumour, distrust, fear and non-compliant behaviour that can contribute to the rapid transmission of a disease.

> People don't resist change. They resist being changed.

The key to effective rumour control is for an agency to have the capacity to perform three functions: (1) rumour identification; (2) rumour investigation; and (3) rumour correction (Burgess and Maiese 2004).

## Rumour identification

A mechanism is needed for determining what rumours are actually circulating. The first step, rumour identification, requires the support of people who are in a position to hear the latest rumours in the community. In general, these are people who are working at the community level (rumour reporters) and that have been provided with training so that they understand how misinformation can drive the cycle of rumour. A means of feedback of new rumours to an agency

---

## BOX 9.2: Using social media to identify rumours

A semi-automatic labelling of tweets and crowdsourcing can be used as a system to identify rumours. To understand and evaluate a rumour, it is often necessary to see multiple posts about that same rumour. A rumour is rarely captured by a single social media post and a large number of distinct tweets, all discussing a single topic, must therefore be collected and analysed.

Rumours transmitted through social media can be broadly classified into the following categories:

- Unsubstantiated information/speculation: A social media post that discusses information that is uncertain or is unsubstantiated.
- Disputed/controversial information: A post that disputes information provided in another post, article, image or video.
- Misinformation/disinformation: A post that contains false information, misrepresents information or quotes out of context.
- Reporting: A post that reports the occurrence of an event and supplies a secondary source, for example a hyperlinked news article.
- Linked dispute: A post that attempts to deny a rumour, possibly in the form or a direct reply to a user. Like reports, corrections often supply a secondary supporting source of evidence.
- Opinionated: A post that expresses the author's opinion.

In practice, it can be difficult to collect and separately identify all classes of rumour-related tweets and, in particular, those containing controversial information can be subject to higher levels of disagreement between assessors (McCreadie et al. 2015).

---

is necessary; for example, social networks such as Twitter have the potential to automatically identify rumours in real time or more traditional methods can be used such as daily briefing meetings.

## Rumour investigation

An effective strategy is needed for determining which rumours are true and which are false. The next phase of the rumour control process, rumour investigation, requires a workable mechanism determining the truthfulness of rumours. Rumour investigators (who may be the same people as the rumour reporters), help determine, from the community perspective, the accuracy of rumours. Significant people in the community, such as school teachers or health workers, are systematically contacted to investigate the latest rumours. When these intermediaries hear a story that they think is likely to be untrue, they can initiate an investigation to try to determine whether the rumour is accurate. Rumour investigators must be able to clearly acknowledge cases in which they are unable to determine the reliability of the source of the rumour. Although there will be cases were the practices of secrecy make reliable rumour checking difficult, there will also be many cases in which incorrect rumours can be partially corrected. The rumour investigators, for example, can be part of a committee made up of people from different agencies that meet periodically to exchange information about current rumours at the local or district level.

## Rumour correction

A mechanism is needed for correcting inaccurate rumours and replacing them with reliable information. This is called counter messaging and part of the third phase of rumour control, rumour correction. The rumour investigators use a reliable mechanism for promptly reporting their findings to the agency which is then communicated to the managers of the outbreak response. In cases when there is no agreement on what has happened, they should report what is known, what is not known, what is still being investigated and any differing interpretations of the facts. When an investigation determines that the rumour is not true, then a plan for correcting the error should be initiated. The success of this plan depends upon the credibility of the information and the ability to communicate the correction widely, effectively and quickly. People that want a reliable information source can be instructed to call a centralised telephone number to find out whether a rumour they have heard is true or not. The rumour hotline allows for direct, immediate communication about the current situation.

## RESISTANCE AND CONFLICT RESOLUTION

Community resistance can be a disruptive feature of a disease outbreak by taking attention away from important issues, by dividing communities and by undermining the positions of the different stakeholders. However, if managed correctly conflict can be a positive ingredient by resolving disputes, helping to release emotions and anxieties and helping communities to address sensitive issues, while simultaneously improving co-operation. Agencies can play an important role in resolving resistance by assessing the situation, being a good listener and inviting partner participation to clarify areas of conflict (Rashid 2012).

Conflict resolution can be used as a method to facilitate the peaceful ending of community resistance by actively communicating information about conflicting perspectives and by engaging people in a collective process of negotiation (Forsyth 2009). This is because the beginnings of conflict are often caused by poor communication between different stakeholders, weak local leadership, internal struggles to gain access to limited resources, disagreements between communities and agencies and an uncertainty about their role in the outbreak response. In conflict situations, those with the control can try to dominate and this can make it difficult to reach a negotiated agreement that is satisfactory to all parties. Those who are in a less powerful position have two main options: (1) to resist by increasing their own resources, organisation and mobilisation and using this in tactics of non-compliance and resistance or (2) to induce those with more power to use it benevolently and to be sympathetic to the inequality of those with less power (Coleman 2000). To enable people to gain more power over option 1 or to be in a better position to negotiate in option 2 requires an approach to resolve conflict. This can include providing training for conflict management, developing communication tools to better disseminate information, using listening to clarify understanding or providing a facilitated dialogue to map and resolve issues.

> Conflict can be resolved in our everyday work by being good listeners and inviting people to simply clarify any issues of concern.

Conflict resolution does not have to be a specialist area of work, especially when the issue of disagreement is not complicated and can often be resolved by a simple clarification and discussion of the main concerns. The conflict resolution can be facilitated by the health promoter using simple, participatory exercises that can be used to help, by mapping the main questions held between the different stakeholders involved and then by developing strategies to address each relevant concern.

## BOX 9.3: An exercise to resolve conflict

To carry out this exercise the health promoter should have some prior knowledge about the key questions that will be asked and some of the solutions that can be discussed. This will help the health promoter to focus the discussion on the practical and not on the personal points. The health promoter should be able to first define the issues of the conflict in neutral terms that all participants can agree upon as follows:

1. The participants are asked to construct a list of key questions about the conflict, the potential solutions to the questions.
2. The participants and the health promoter next identify sources of the information regarding each of the key questions (e.g. websites, local leaders, government officials) that are necessary to move into a problem-solving stage.
3. The participants are asked to prepare a summary of the conflict by comparing each question with a possible solution and a source of information. This can be usefully summarised in a table.
4. After a period of discussion between the different parties the table can be rewritten to highlight how major changes in one conflict alters over time as circumstances change.

It is necessary to note that this type of a problem-solving exercise is not a negotiation but is a commitment to further analysis and discussion (Mitchell and Banks 1998).

# MILITARY COORDINATION

Military coordination refers to the use of military capabilities to help address a disease outbreak. The 2014 Ebola outbreak revealed that in the absence of robust health systems at the national level and a rapid humanitarian response at the international level, civil-military co-operation can be decisive. The military intervention provides essential skills and capabilities that can be used to leverage domestic military and civilian forces to productively engage in the response. The response deployed thousands of international military personnel to help contain the spread of the disease, mostly UK and US military forces, that were primarily used to construct treatment units and for the training of local health workers (Kamradt-Scott et al. 2015). Military involvement is often based on historic patterns of occupation and this can create distrust in the local population because it seems to be a repeat of patterns of oppression. The multi-national nature of a military coordination can help to alleviate concerns and integrate small units of trusted regional forces. In Liberia and Sierra Leone, the presence of American and British troops helped give the outbreak response some authority. In contrast, Guinea did not have support from a foreign military and, because of its history, did not deploy its own army. However, the gendarme force, which is distinct from the army, was integrated into the response to assist with establishing the initial system of coordination (Dhillon and Kelly 2015).

> Clear statements of military activities in the disease outbreak can help to alleviate community concerns.

## BOX 9.4: Using the short message service in areas of conflict

The security situation in parts of Somalia is volatile and directly impacts on healthcare delivery including the control of disease outbreaks such as the poliovirus as well as on routine immunisation programmes, resulting in low coverage. Armed conflict and clan clashes reduce access for house-to-house, campaign-based activities and the movement of health workers, especially remote to households, areas inaccessible due to insurgency, coastal regions where piracy is an issue and among nomadic groups. The large number of un-vaccinated children (estimated at 1 million) posed a real risk for the re-emergence of a polio outbreak. Communicating with families in the affected districts to encourage them to visit the nearest health facility for the vaccination of their children was identified through radio and short message service platforms. The short message service platform was delivered as an interactive combination of questions and messages and an effective way of reducing the security risks to health workers (Birungi et al. 2016).

The military coordination in an emergency deployment, in conjunction with the activation of the local national defence forces, can be a new experience in some countries. Some police and military units are regarded as trustworthy and community self-defence networks may be mobilised as well as ex-combatants that remain in place from previous conflicts. Military personnel may receive culturally related pre-deployment training. However, most will arrive in-country unaware of how to interact with communities and how much they are negatively perceived by the local population. Training for military personnel is therefore required to boost their preparedness, build awareness, and to ensure a reciprocal understanding of appropriate roles and responsibilities, specifically in the health sector, and what they cannot or should not do in-country (Kamradt-Scott et al. 2015).

A disease outbreak can quickly develop to overreach the capacity of local police and military units especially when the previous experience has been limited to providing support to healthcare facilities. The result is a necessity to deploy military forces to control potential civil unrest. The role and responsibilities of the military in specific locations such as in clinics and government buildings should be communicated to the public. Contact information should also be provided to the public for reporting perceived abuses by the military to avoid confrontation with communities, disseminated by government and non-government agencies in collaboration with the military response. This is best achieved using both a local contact person and a military contact facilitated through an open public discussion, for example, community meetings, about what will happen when the military forces are on the ground and how to report any incidents (George Washington University 2014).

## COMMUNITY QUARANTINES

One way to decrease the transmission rate of infectious diseases is to recognise the effects of interactions within hubs (or groups) of infected individuals and other interactions within discrete hubs of susceptible individuals. Despite the low interaction between discrete hubs, the disease can jump to and spread in a susceptible hub via a single interaction with an infected hub. Infection rates can be reduced if interactions between individuals within infected hubs are eliminated, but they can be even more drastically reduced if the main focus is on the prevention of transmission jumps between hubs (Watts 2003). An example of the implementation of this type on an initiative is the use of community quarantines in controlling infectious diseases.

Quarantine interventions can be applied as the context of an outbreak changes. In Sierra Leone, for example, a household was quarantined if a member of the family was confirmed to be infected by the Ebola virus. They remained in quarantine for 21 days if there were no new symptoms. In Liberia, this approach was different and included any contact – suspected, probable or confirmed. A suspected case is any person, alive or dead, who has (or had) sudden onset of high fever and had contact with a suspected, probable or confirmed Ebola case, or a dead or sick animal or any person with sudden onset of high fever and at least three of the following symptoms: headache; vomiting; anorexia/loss of appetite; diarrhoea; lethargy; stomach pain; aching muscles or joints; difficulty swallowing; and breathing difficulties; or any person with unexplained bleeding or any sudden, unexplained death. A probable case is any suspected case evaluated by a clinician or any person who died from 'suspected' Ebola and had an epidemiological link to a confirmed case but was not tested and did not have laboratory confirmation of the disease. A confirmed case is a probable or suspected case is classified as confirmed when a sample from that person tests positive for Ebola in the laboratory (World Health Organization 2014a).

A quarantine differs from isolation. All suspected and probable cases are immediately isolated until they receive results from a laboratory test. In Sierra Leone as the outbreak continued, more communities and villages were quarantined. By December 2014, more than 1 million people in quarantine required food assistance. Movement restrictions helped create the food shortages, contributing to a lack of labour, trading and commodities. However, throughout this period people continued to violate quarantines in search of basic provisions. Households frequently did not receive food packages within 24 hours of being placed under a quarantine. Quarantine can produce experiences of a lower household income, and this leads to critical levels of food insecurity, especially when it interferes with the harvest or the planting season. Food should be distributed to people once a week during the 21 days of quarantine, but in many cases this did not happen (ACAPS 2015). The use of individual, household and community quarantines as a security strategy during an outbreak has been criticised for causing panic and resistance; however, it is a vital tool to prevent the spread of infection and to facilitate contact tracing (Laverack and Manoncourt 2015).

## Community-led quarantines

Raising the awareness of communities about the benefits of quarantines and the role that they can play in stopping the outbreak is essential. Community-led quarantines are not problematic if the timely and reliable delivery of resources, such as food and water, are received by the person or household being detained.

### BOX 9.5: Minimising quarantine violations in Liberia

In Liberia, quarantines were most effective at the community level, coordinated by local people and religious leaders. This was crucial to minimising violations of the quarantine as well as to the tracing of contacts and of new cases. There were variations in how communities implemented the quarantine; for example, some communities denied the quarantined contacts access to water and basic provisions, whereas other communities provided water and food independently. The availability of services to remove bodies safely and to train contact tracers were also important to deter quarantine violations. The shift from denial to acceptance of the existence or causes of Ebola was another major factor in promoting compliance with quarantines. As more of the population witnessed the personal impact of the disease first-hand, such as by having relatives who became infected or died, the denial of its existence and resistance to the international response decreased (ACAPS 2015).

Community-led quarantines are important in the success of outbreak responses.

Community-led quarantines have proven to be an important factor, especially when they were led by village and faith leaders, and helped to minimise quarantine violations, as well as to trace new contacts and cases. The reliable delivery of resources was also an essential part of building community-led quarantines including food, water, money and information (Sahr Sahidn 2015).

## VIOLENCE AND PROTESTS

Conflict and disease outbreaks interact, often feeding off each other, to worsen the situation because (1) a disease outbreak can create conflict through instability, weakening economic capacity through the depletion of resources provided to halt the outbreak and instilling fear in the population that the disease may spread to them; and (2) conflict can further create the spread of the disease through the geographic movement of infected individuals, as well as through preventing efforts to control the outbreak.

Violence against health professionals was seen as early as April 2015 in Guinea when a crowd attacked an Ebola isolation centre and threw rocks at aid workers, stemming from their fear of the disease. In another community, the bodies of eight health workers and journalists were found after they went missing during a case investigation in a remote area. The residents attacked the group believing they were trying to bring Ebola to their village (*Huffington Post*, 18 September 2014). On 1 September 2015, hundreds of youth in Liberia protested about the secret burial of suspected cases. They dug up the bodies to move them out of the area, which exposed individuals to a higher risk of infection, as the dead bodies were highly infectious. The number of riots and protests related to the outbreak, as well as instances of violence against civilians, increased. Another violent incident occurred on 17 September 2015, when after attacking aid workers, villagers in Guinea erected barricades and destroyed a bridge to intentionally block access to their town because they believed the outsiders were coming with the Ebola disease (Armed Conflict Location and Event Data Project 2014).

An example of using security measures to avoid violence and protests while working to control the spread of an infectious disease was the National 'Getting To Zero' Ebola Campaign in Sierra Leone started on 27 March until 25 April 2015. Getting To Zero was intended to ensure that Sierra Leone had no Ebola cases for 42 days. The objective was to reinvigorate the fight against Ebola, address the issue of complacency, and help communities to keep up safe practices. The agency focus was on active case finding and vigilance such as using neighbourhood watch approaches. For the first 3 days of the campaign, everyone was instructed to stay at home. No passes to travel were issued and security personnel checked ID cards and passports. However, even during the high-profile security intervention exceptions had to be made for healthcare workers at public and private facilities, private security companies and some commercial vehicles to transport people to and from religious services. The strict measures and the deployment of military and security forces helped to prevent crime and violence and to enforce compliance with during the curfew (Ministry of Health 2015).

## CROSS-BORDER ISSUES

In many countries, international borders are considered to be porous and artificially separating already closely interwoven communities linked by common languages, ethnicity, cultural traditions and access to markets. A preliminary analysis of the decision to close international borders between Guinea and Liberia, for example, concluded the following:

- Communities are closely linked by common vernacular languages, ethnicity, cultural traditions for marriage and burial, intermarriage, access to schools, clinics, churches, weekly markets.
- Most foot/bicycle traffic and illegal border crossings are destined for proximate communities along borders rather than the deep interior.
- Border control is useless for the short-distance migration and only community engagement and surveillance will provide protection.
- Radio and churches were the most important source of information.
- The role of the village chief in controlling cross-border movement is critical and when properly engaged and committed, control measures were better organised and more rigorous (Wolff 2015).

The cross-border movement of people is inevitable and although the closing of official border crossings can prevent motor vehicle traffic, foot and bicycle traffic continues and may even increase in remote areas, acting as a potential source of disease transmission (Laverack and Manoncourt 2015).

> Community management of cross-border movement includes activities that are crucial to a successful response such as community policing and contact tracing.

Action involving the Ministry of Interior, the Police and Gendarmerie and other governmental partners in border management in Mauritania and Senegal in West Africa has provided practical solutions. Mauritania and Senegal share an 850-km border running the length of the Senegal River which people cross every

> **BOX 9.6: Strengthening border surveillance between Ebola-affected countries**
>
> Cross-border surveillance was a key component in the response to the Ebola outbreak in West Africa. Border Coordination Groups, often chaired by the Ministry of Health, were established to strengthen surveillance and included members from the Bureau of Immigration, Police, United Nations Mission for Ebola Emergency Response, World Health Organization, Centers for Disease Control and Prevention, International Organization for Migration, United Nations Children's Fund, key non-government organisations and Office for the Coordination of Humanitarian Affairs. A series of measures were facilitated by the Border Coordination Groups, including the enforcement of quarantines in border communities, the training of key officials at border crossing points, standard operating procedures for health screening, notification and the referral of cases and equipping the crossing points with facilities for the isolation of suspected cases. The governments of Guinea and Sierra Leone signed a memorandum of understanding providing for a national-level supervision of cross-border interventions, information sharing and a focus on community ownership. Health promotion campaigns in hotspot border areas were used to maintain vigilance and promote preventative measures such as hand-washing and safe burials and were supported by the distribution of hygiene kits (OCHA 2015).

day for economic, family or social reasons. There is no system in place to facilitate the efficient and secure cross-border movement of people. A feasibility study looked at three border management options. The first option involved border residents giving their identity card to Mauritanian border officers, who would keep it until the resident re-crossed the border to return to Senegal. The second option would involve the creation of a dedicated border resident identity card. The third option would use pre-registered biometric information to enable residents to enter and leave the Mauritanian territory (IOM 2015). These top-down solutions require significant involvement of security forces and an alternative is to allow communities to manage the cross-border movement of people in their locality either in collaboration with authorities or independent of all top-down measures.

## Community management of cross-border movement

Strong community engagement is recognised as a key element in all cross-border prevention strategies. Cross-border transmission is the way in which many diseases are introduced into another country and the most likely route for a reintroduction as long as an outbreak continues in a region. However, communities can be mobilised to help prevent the transmission of a disease as well as to control and monitor cross-border movement.

---

**BOX 9.7: Community management of cross-border movement in Sierra Leone**

Koinadugu is the one of the few districts in Sierra Leone that did not record a case of Ebola during the early stages of the outbreak. Koinadugu is in the Northern Province and is the largest district in Sierra Leone, with an ethnically diverse population estimated at 265,765. The district borders Bombali on the west, Tonkolili district to the southwest, Kono district to the south and the Republic of Guinea to northeast. Diamond mining and agriculture are the main economic activities and the main religion is Islam, with more than 85% of the population. In June 2014 people came together to form a task force including politicians, paramount chiefs, local community leaders, doctors and influential women. These people started meeting regularly and made a pledge that they would not allow their community to become infected with the virus. People walked long distances to come to meetings and no incentives were given, but people had a real conviction to protect their communities. People in the district respected and listened to their leaders. They collectively decided that no stranger would be allowed into the district without first checking with the chief or village headman. Taxi drivers were encouraged to transport people only within the district and pledged not to travel outside the district. The movement of traders and market people outside the district was also limited. A marketplace intelligence committee was used to prevent traders from taking advantage of the limited trading movement. A joint team of military, police, medical and youth groups helped to monitor entry and exit points in and out of the district. People entering the district were subjected to a thorough screening process to determine their status before they were allowed to travel further (World Health Organization 2015b).

---

A systematic community management approach is feasible to record travel histories, to trace contacts and to isolate suspected cases and then to notify the authorities. The key actors are village chiefs, community volunteers and local health facilities where standards of basic infection, prevention and control can be enforced. For example, engaging with village chiefs in cross-border control is critical to organise patrols of the boundaries of their villages, to keep outsiders away and to record people's movements. To promote the involvement of communities in controlling cross-border movement a rapid assessment protocol for activities can be developed and an analysis plan based on the assessment used to summarise any necessary actions (Wolff 2015).

# 10

# The post-outbreak and emergency response

**KEY POINTS**

- After every large-scale response, there is the hope that lessons in regard to community engagement will be learned, but this is seldom realised.
- The donor community is better able than ever before to coordinate a global response, but it must also support existing health systems in at-risk, low-income countries.
- Self-help groups enable people to move forward to broader concerns, build networks and have greater influence by working together with other people.
- Survivors can sometimes offer a valuable role by providing support in high-risk, infectious situations without infecting themselves or others.
- The health promoter can play an important role by listening to community members and feeding their concerns back to healthcare providers about how services can be improved.

Disease outbreaks can lead to a breakdown in health systems and can deny people access to healthcare, vaccines and essential medicines. The result is an increase in mortality and morbidity from, for example, preventable communicable diseases. After conflict in the Democratic Republic of Congo, most deaths were due to preventable conditions, especially in children under the age of 5 years, and accounted for more than 45% of all deaths caused by fever, malaria and diarrhoea (Coghlan et al. 2006). The Ebola outbreak in West Africa largely overwhelmed the healthcare system, making it difficult to then treat many endemic communicable diseases. One study estimated that if malaria care ceased as a result of the Ebola outbreak, untreated cases of malaria would have increased by 45% in Guinea, 88% in Sierra Leone and 140% in Liberia in 2014. This increase is equivalent to 3.5 million additional untreated cases, with approximately 10,900 additional malaria-attributable deaths. The findings suggest that untreated malaria cases, as a result of reduced healthcare capacity, probably contributed as substantially to morbidity as did the Ebola outbreak (Walker et al. 2015). Another study suggested there could have been a rise of more than 100,000 measles and predicted that the increase would advance from 127,000 at the start of the Ebola outbreak in 2014 to 227,000 after 18 months. This would result in an additional 5000–16,000 measles deaths, potentially more than the actual number of reported Ebola deaths, largely caused by an interruption in immunisation programmes. The study also estimated that 1,129,376 children aged between 9 months and 5 years were unvaccinated, compared with 778,000 before the outbreak (Roberts 2015).

Disease outbreaks can be addressed through the deployment of simultaneous public health and universal healthcare interventions. The relaunching of health services following an outbreak is an urgent priority because children have missed vaccinations, patients have their treatment interrupted and pregnant women require a safe place to deliver. However, the post-outbreak interventions that take place must also build capacity to improve the ability of human resources to detect, investigate and address new outbreaks.

> After every large-scale response, there is the hope that lessons in regard to community engagement will be learned, but this is seldom realised.

Human resources for health addresses the planning, development, performance, management and staff retention for the healthcare sector. The reasons for health worker shortages in sub-Saharan Africa, where outbreaks frequently occur, have been attributed to investment shortfalls in pre-service training, international migration and premature retirement. In 2005, it was estimated that 25% of all doctors and 5% of all nurses trained in sub-Saharan Africa had emigrated to work in Organisation for Economic Co-operation and Development member countries (World Health Organization 2006b). Technological advances and consumer expectations can also dramatically shift demands on the health workforce to seek opportunities and job security in other labour markets, intensifying professional concentrations in urban areas and in wealthier countries. This has created a workforce crisis in countries that are vulnerable to disease outbreaks characterised by severe staff shortages, inappropriate skill mixes and gaps in service delivery (World Health Organization 2006a). The international aid community must therefore engage with those countries that lack the human resource capacity to respond to disease outbreaks (MSF 2015).

> The donor community is better able than ever before to coordinate a global response, but it must also support existing health systems in at-risk, low-income countries.

Universal healthcare refers to a health system organised around providing a specified package of benefits to all citizens and is an essential long-term goal in the post-outbreak response. The aim is to provide financial risk protection, improved access to health services and improved health outcomes. Universal healthcare is not a one-size-fits-all concept, nor does it imply coverage for all people for all health needs (World Health Organization 2010). The aim is to create resilient health systems that are well equipped and staffed and allow locally managed resources to be fully utilised and are therefore not dependent on donated goods and services (Wilkinson and Leach 2014). A Basic Package of Health Services was developed in Afghanistan by using a mixed model of funding to deliver post-conflict and manageable services, as explained in the box below.

---

### BOX 10.1: The Basic Package of Health Services, Afghanistan

The Basic Package of Health Services was developed in 2005 by the Ministry of Public Health of Afghanistan to deliver affordable and manageable interventions in areas of post-conflict. The Basic Package of Health Services was designed to cover maternal and newborn health, immunisation, the control of communicable diseases and nutrition. Mental health and the management of disabilities were also given a priority. The Ministry of Public Health of Afghanistan took on a supervisory role and employed non-government organisations to deliver the Basic Package of Health Services interventions, often using a community-based approach. In the short term, this approach was relatively effective; for example, the number of functioning health centres increased, access to health services increased as did the coverage of vaccinations. Areas of conflict or where conflict had resumed have demonstrated significantly lower levels of access and coverage in Afghanistan (Waldman and Kruk 2011).

---

## COMMUNITY RESILIENCE

Resilience can be defined as the capacity of individuals, families, communities, systems and institutions to anticipate, withstand and/or engage with catastrophic events (Almedom and Tumwine 2008). Community resilience uses local assets to allow people to better cope in a disease outbreak and complements the response to help make the transition from an emergency to longer term development. Communities can spontaneously help one another in times of crisis, and those that have planned and prepared for a health emergency are better able to cope and to recover more quickly. This can also contribute to the resilience of a public health system by strengthening existing strengths before a disease outbreak. For example, local resilience forums in the UK meet regularly to discuss emergency preparedness tailored to reflect local authority priorities and capabilities.

## BOX 10.2: Disaster preparedness in the Philippines

The "Community-Based Disaster Risk Management and Local Governance" was implemented in the city of Dagupan, north of Manila, on Luzon Island in northern Philippines. The purpose was to build governmental, organisational and community skills for better risk management. This was achieved through better coordination, capacity building and training. Grants for disaster risk management and climate change adaptation were also provided to encourage local action. In particular, the project provided an opportunity for city officials to go to urban communities and to train on Community-Based Disaster Risk Management. Disaster Coordinating Councils helped develop community disaster risk reduction plans and community early warning and evacuation plans. Open dialogues also allowed members of vulnerable communities to voice their grievances to the city officials, including to the city mayor, leading to several joint disaster mitigation activities. For example, earthquake and evacuation drills were carried out, covering 55,000 school students and teachers (Center for Disaster Preparedness 2015).

The membership is comprised of relevant services including fire and police, health bodies and government agencies such as the Environment Agency and representatives from neighbouring resilience forums and is often chaired by the chief executive of a high-level responder agency such as an emergency service. The local forums are a multidisciplinary team that is formed to develop practical plans in advance of a disease outbreak or emergency (Lewis 2016).

The national level response to a disease outbreak can have negative consequences on community resilience because the highly centralised command structure, although advantageous for the rapid delivery of resources at scale, is not conducive to identifying and responding to local needs. A failure to appreciate and engage with local priorities can lead to an ineffective response effort that can be further hindered by community resistance and the inefficient delivery of services and resources (Richards 2015).

## THE ROLE OF HEALTH PROMOTION IN THE POST-OUTBREAK RESPONSE

The post-outbreak response is an important period to improve health and to aid recovery and rehabilitation within society. Health promotion has an important role in increasing awareness about available facilities and to promote participation in using services such as vaccination, counselling and welfare initiatives. Health promotion can help to mobilise communities to assist with rehabilitation services for people with disabilities associated with the disease outbreak. Health promotion can also help to build social support networks for the survivors of an outbreak and to counter stigma and isolation.

## Addressing stigma and social isolation

After recovering from an infectious disease, people can suffer stigma and social isolation. Many survivors prefer to stay anonymous to avoid being stigmatised by other people, even by their own family and community. Stigmatisation brands someone as being different in ways that can result in discrimination, loss of status and social exclusion. For example, the high mortality rate of Ebola led to survivors being associated with special powers, making it difficult for them to integrate back into their communities. Other people who were ill, the family or households of those under quarantine and those regularly in contact with patients such as health workers were also susceptible to stigma. One knowledge, attitude and practice survey in Sierra Leone, covering 1413 households, confirmed that Ebola survivors faced high levels of stigma and discrimination. This undermined their ability to recover their livelihoods and to re-continue their lives. The survey indicated that 96% people reported a discriminatory attitude towards survivors, 76% said that they would not welcome someone back into their community and 9% would keep the information secret if a family member contracted Ebola (UNICEF 2015c). Addressing the stigma associated with a disease is critical for people to regain their dignity and livelihoods.

People caught in the cycle of high-risk conditions and poor social support are less likely to be active in self-help groups concerned with improving their situation. This can reinforce their sense of isolation and self-blame, compounding the negative experiences and physical symptoms affecting the person's social, physical and mental well-being. Social well-being includes interpersonal relationships as well as wider social issues such as marital satisfaction and community cohesion. The role of relationships, family support and a person's status at work are important to feelings of social well-being as these help to increase a sense of inclusion, connectedness and self-esteem. Physical well-being is concerned with concepts such as the proper functioning of the body, biological normality and the capacity to perform tasks such that an individual is physically fit and unimpaired. Mental well-being involves concepts such as self-efficacy and social inclusion and is the ability of people to adapt to their environment and the society in which they function (Walker and Marie 2011).

Once an outbreak has become established, stigmatisation can be more socially embedded; for example, stigma has reduced significantly in regard to HIV and there has been a normalisation of the disease and its associated risks. The first step to addressing stigma is to identify the nature of, and factors influencing, relationships between those associated with the disease and the rest of society. The two most effective interventions to de-stigmatise a disease are (1) to improve survival and knowledge about the ability to survive and (2) to prevent negative economic consequences of those suffering from the disease. In the absence of a treatment, addressing stigma requires a reduction in the social isolation and the negative perceptions of those associated with the disease. Efforts to de-stigmatise Ebola, for example, aimed to improve the physical, economic and social well-being as well as the social visibility of those groups associated with the disease. Providing households under quarantine with compensation or a 'de-stigmatisation kit' that ensured access to a phone, phone credit and a cash transfer to cover the cost of food mitigated some of the socially isolating effects and negative economic consequences. It also transformed the perception of some quarantined households into opportunities for their neighbours (Ebola Response Anthropology Platform 2014).

## Self-help groups

Self-help groups organise around a specific personal concern such as rehabilitation after a period of poor health. Group members have a shared interest, are supportive of one another and often manage the group meetings themselves (Laverack 2009). Self-help is often a self-guided improvement, economically, intellectually, or emotionally, either face to face or through the Internet to provide a greater sense of belonging. Self-help groups can be used to learn about health problems and to gain specific skills through training and peer support. The involvement in, and the development of, self-help groups is an important approach in health promotion because they can be the starting point for collective action. This locale also provides an opportunity for the health promoter to assist in support activities, for example, to help the mothers of newborn babies affected by microcephaly to receive financial and others resources. A needs assessment is sometimes necessary to identify the common concerns of the group members, the solutions and actions to resolve their concerns. When these skills do not exist or are weak, the role of the health promoter is to assist the group to make an assessment. Self-help groups often have limited resources, and their small size can lead to them being absorbed into the policy-making process, thus losing their purpose and identity unless they are able to grow and develop into broader community-based organisations (Allsop et al. 2004).

> Self-help groups enable people to move forward to broader concerns, build networks and have greater influence by working together with other people.

## WORKING WITH POST-OUTBREAK SURVIVORS

The survivors of disease outbreaks face significant life changes, having sometimes lost their relatives, friends and livelihoods. This is compounded by fractured social networks in an environment, often characterised with high levels of poverty and food insecurity. Providing psychosocial support to survivors is an important element in supporting resilience in rebuilding their lives, including identifying any serious mental health issues and working in conjunction with a referral system for those people who require specialised care (Dalling and Bangura 2014).

Health facilities in West Africa presented survivors with a certificate and some material support at the point of discharge. However, Ebola survivors then faced physical, economic and social barriers to rebuilding their lives, including return-ing to their own communities. The ability of survivors to re-integrate back into their communities was hindered by rumours that they were still infectious, poor physical health and a reduced economic situation. Some survivors were provided with psychosocial support to ensure that they adhered to infection control prac-tices. In other cases, a unique ID card was given to survivors to record their progress through each stage of re-integration. Re-integration cards were first used in Sierra Leone for disarmament, demobilisation and the re-integration of ex-combatants showing their engagement in civic duties and were a highly valued symbol of their reintegration into society. The programme highlighted the need for a robust identification of patients to prevent fraudulent claimants, the illegal selling of ID cards, transparent systems for distributing material and financial support and allowing the wider community to benefit from the support to avoid conflict (Kamradt-Scott et al. 2015).

Re-integration begins when the patient moves into the health facility conva-lescent area and then when they have tested negative for the disease and are ready for discharge. Next, the survivor makes a commitment to adhere to a code of practice that is appropriate behaviour for their recovery. The community also pledges to provide support, welcome the survivor back and participate with the survivor in communal social activities. The supporting organisation commits to provide financial and material compensation to the survivor and to the commu-nity. A health promoter can accompany the survivor back to their community to answer questions and to offer an endorsement as an 'expert' person to commu-nity leaders. The issue of a public statement as a decision by the significant part of the community shows that a sufficient number of people have decided, on moral grounds, not to stigmatise or isolate the survivor (Ebola Response Anthropology Platform 2014a). This is a health promotion approach called 'moral suasion' and an act of trying to use moral principles to influence individuals and groups to change their practices, beliefs and actions (Laverack 2013a).

## SURVIVOR NETWORKS

A network is a structure of relationships that in turn are the building blocks of interaction and experience, mapping the connections that individuals have to one another (Pescosolido 1991) and the impact that it has on people's lives (White 1992). Social networks offer many people the opportunity to strengthen the relationships in their lives and can be used to spread positive health behav-iours because people's perceptions of their own risk of illness may depend on the people around them (Christakis and Fowler 2007). Trust, social norms of reciprocity reside in relationships and in the social networks in which they participate. Active participation within social networks builds cohesiveness between individuals and is important to mobilise and create the resources necessary to support collective action.

There are estimated to be more than 10,000 survivors of the Ebola virus disease in West Africa (World Health Organization 2016), of which 4500 survivors have been registered and organised to form support networks. Survivor networks can

> ## BOX 10.3: Survivor networks in Sierra Leone
>
> More than 400 Ebola survivors met in Sierra Leone's Bombali District to share their experiences and to discuss issues of stigma and discrimination. This meeting created a network for survivors and was organised by the Ministry of Social Welfare, Gender and Children's Affairs to help survivors to continue their recovery. The network was able to promote approaches that its members had identified as working well in addressing stigma. For example, radio broadcasts had proven to be one of the most effective ways of reaching communities through messages broadcast on 62 radio stations supported by one-on-one discussions at the household level to help raise the awareness of the needs of survivors (UNICEF 2014)

be a strategic population for the post-outbreak response through assisting with safe and dignified burials, caring for the sick and orphaned children, providing community outreach and donating blood.

Survivors can sometimes offer a valuable role by providing support in high-risk, infectious situations without infecting themselves or others.

## SURVIVOR INCLUSION IN BLOOD AND PLASMA DONATIONS

Verified Ebola survivors (VES) that were willing to participate in ongoing whole blood and plasma donor programmes were a potential resource in the post-outbreak response. Eligible VES had to be in good health and be at least 2 months after a second negative test from a health facility. Working with VES can occur in two stages for the identification, recruitment, maintenance and retention of a network of VES (see Figure 10.1). Stage 1 involves the identification, recruitment, health check and a verification of survivors onto the convalescent plasma intervention. It also involves the establishment of a blood and plasma donor network to maintain contact with the VES. A package of support is introduced during Stage 1 that includes regular health screening and treatment at a health facility, counselling, assistance to integrate into society and material support. Stage 2 involves informed consent from the donor and whole blood donation or plasmapheresis, the continuation of the blood and plasma donor network and an expansion of its activities to address VES needs.

### Preparation

A standard operational procedure including training materials and information sheets allows peer educators and recruiters to quickly build a dialogue with VES.

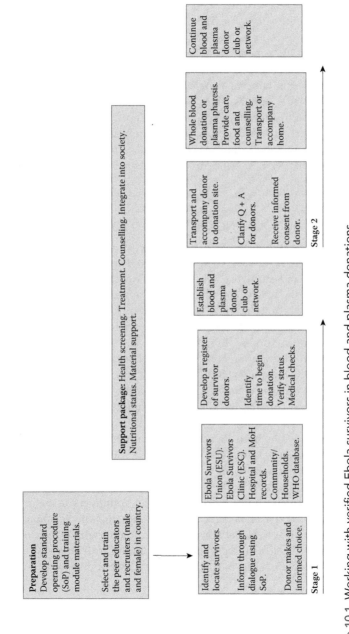

Figure 10.1 Working with verified Ebola survivors in blood and plasma donations.

The training is carried out over 1 day to strengthen knowledge and communication skills for conversations about becoming a donor. The use of peer educators is an established approach (UNICEF 2013) in which lay persons are felt to be in the best position to encourage behaviour change in others rather than using health workers. This is especially important in cross-cultural and sensitive contexts such as working with survivors. The peer education process is initiated by the investigators who recruit members of the 'target' community to serve as educators and recruiters. These people are typically about the same age as the VES, may be survivors themselves and consist of both males and females. The intention of peer education is that familiar people, giving locally relevant and meaningful suggestions, in a local language and taking account of the local context, will be more likely to recruit. They may work alongside the health workers, run activities on their own, or actually take the lead in organising and implementing activities for the VES, such as blood and plasma donor clubs. Importantly, the peer educators act as a link between the survivors and the blood donation agency.

## Stage 1

### IDENTIFYING AND LOCATING THE VERIFIED EBOLA SURVIVORS

The peer educators and recruiters firstly engage with established networks and associations to contact the survivors, for example, through the survivors' unions and associations and survivors' clinics. These settings provide opportunities to contact numerous survivors and also act as a means to identify others with whom the participants are familiar including family and friends. This type of a 'snow-balling' recruitment process has the potential to lead to many new contacts for the identification of VES. These contacts may be located in both rural communities and in urban centres. For peer educators and recruiters visiting rural communities, it is important that they are already a member of this community to avoid any risk of conflict. Survivors can also be identified and located at hospitals where they congregate, faith-based organisations and through Ministry of Health records.

Once a survivor has been identified and located, the peer educators and recruiters will develop a dialogue by using the standard operational procedure to provide information and to clarify any concerns that the person may have about donating blood and plasma. The purpose is to allow the survivor to make an informed choice before he or she volunteers to be a potential donor. Once the survivor has agreed to be a donor, it is the normal procedure to ascertain when he or she is ready to donate, to refer him or her for a medical examination (physical and psychological) and to verify his or her status as a survivor through a health centre or personal discharge records.

### THE SUPPORT PACKAGE

The VES can receive a support package to assist in recovery and re-integration back into society. The support package will include regular health screening, treatment and the monitoring of nutritional status at a health facility, counselling and assistance to integrate into society through employment and some material support such as blankets and cooking utensils. The support package is not an incentive to be a donor in the convalescent plasma intervention, but it is a genuine attempt to help survivors to recover.

After Stage 1 is completed, it is important to maintain contact with the VES through a register of their personal details and through establishing a blood and plasma donor club or network. The purpose of the network is to provide survivors with an opportunity to support and help one another, to share experiences and to take part in activities that build their sense of civic pride and help them to reintegrate. Badges and clothing may also be offered to the members of the blood and plasma donor network to emphasise their contribution to the society and to help to reduce stigma.

## Stage 2

### BLOOD AND PLASMA DONATION

The VES should be accompanied and, if necessary, transported to the blood transfusion service facility. The VES should be given the opportunity to clarify any questions that they may still have about donating blood. Once agreed the VES can complete the informed consent form and then proceed with a whole blood donation using standard protocols such as the guidance for National Health Authorities and Blood Transfusion Services (World Health Organization 2014). The blood transfusion service should provide good care, refreshments, counselling and support to the survivors at the time of the donation. Once the process of donation and support has been completed, the VES should be accompanied, or where necessary, transported home. After Stage 2 is completed, it is important to maintain contact with the VES and to continue the activities of the blood and plasma donor network. The network can be used to identify and address the needs of survivors regarding their health, personal relationships and employment issues by supporting and helping one another.

### THE CONTINUATION OF A CONVALESCENT PLASMA PROGRAMME

It is important to retain the donor services of the VES for the future access to whole blood and plasma. The package of support and the donor network which starts in Stage 1 will be an essential aspect of retention and will continue after Stage 2 has been completed. The strategy is an ongoing programme of training, identification, support, donation and retention. It is also important to retain the services of the peer educators and recruiters in the programme and a form of compensation may be provided, for example, some of the benefits of the support package.

## COUNSELLING AND SURVIVOR SUPPORT INITIATIVES

Counselling occurs when a person consults someone else in regard to a problem, conflict or dilemma that is preventing them from living their lives in a way that they would wish to do so (McLeod and McLeod 2011, 1). A common factor in most counselling situations is that the client is emotionally distressed or otherwise in a negative state of mind about something. A critical variable in the style of counselling used is the extent to which the solution to problems is provided by the counsellor or by the client (Dryden and Feltham 1993). To improve counselling, the health promoter can follow a simple procedure of listening, giving advice and obtaining and providing feedback. Listening is an active process focussing on what the individual is saying and if necessary helping the speaker to express his or her feelings or to give an opinion on an issue. When giving advice the health promoter is exerting his or her expertise to persuade others into accepting a prescribed advice, for example, giving a precise instruction such as the self-treatment to ensure their compliance. Obtaining and giving feedback enable the health promoter to clarify what the person wants and that they have understood previous communication or retained skills. This may mean obtaining feedback based on specific information by using closed questions that require short factual (yes/no) answers or based on an open form of questioning to provide fuller answers. Giving feedback is important for the achievement of effective one-to-one communication and in particular positive feedback that reinforces knowledge. The person is encouraged to share his or her concerns, feelings and opinions, but the discussion is directed by the health promoter.

To help overcome discrimination and to support survivors in returning to their own homes, it may be possible to facilitate community discussions and to encourage others to celebrate their return. After the initial return home, the community can be supported by visits from a health promoter to follow up on the well-being of survivors and to provide opportunities for employment in the post-outbreak response, for example, working with the ambulance services, burial teams, surveillance teams or as contact tracers (SMAC 2014).

> The health promoter can play an important role by listening to community members and feeding their concerns back to healthcare providers about how services can be improved.

## BOX 10.4: Ebola survivor stories

The purpose of the exercise is to help survivors to discuss the reasons for delaying or refusing treatment and any stigma or rejection that they have experienced through storytelling. The exercise takes about 30 minutes. To really be impactful, the experiences should be shared by survivors themselves. It is useful to explore different roles within the family, particularly around caretaking, because not everyone is able to care for the sick, and there may be a designated person in the family to do this activity. At the start, ask whether there are any survivors in the group, and the facilitator should make a point of embracing them and telling people you are not afraid of them.

1. Invite the survivor to tell his or her story, but also ask whether anyone knows a survivor. If so, invite that person to tell his or her friend's story.
2. If the conversation is difficult, begin by asking questions about what happened: how do they think they caught Ebola? How did they feel? What did they do when they started to feel symptoms? Why did they go to the treatment centre? What happened at the treatment centre? What happened when they returned home?
3. When the story is finished, ask for a volunteer to describe what the survivor did or did not do that may have contributed to their survival. What are the key lessons for the group? What would you do if that happened to you? How do you think you would feel?
4. The story can open up further discussion on what is happening in treatment centres. Ask the following: What concerns do community members have about the isolation units and treatment centres? What is it like to be a patient? What food and drink do they receive? What happens when they die? Can they have visitors?
5. This story should also raise issues about stigma. Ask the following: Would you buy food from a survivor? Would you share a meal with a survivor? How do you think they feel? (SMAC 2014).

## Health promotion and medical complications

Several medical complications have been reported in survivors of disease outbreaks such as for the Ebola and Zika viruses. The post-Ebola syndrome affects those who have recovered, and symptoms include joint and muscle pain, eye problems, blindness and various neurological problems. Health risks associated with the Zika virus include symptoms of mild fever, skin rash, conjunctivitis, muscle and joint pain, malaise or headache. However, for the women who are infected in the first trimester, there is a chance that their baby will have microcephaly and the virus can also cause Guillain–Barré syndrome, leading to neurological complications. The Zika and Ebola viruses may persist in some body fluids, and survivors often need comprehensive support for the medical and psychosocial challenges that they face and to minimise the risk of continued virus transmission, for example, through sexual contact (World Health Organization 2016).

Health promotion activities for medical complications in survivors include the following:

- Counselling advice in survivor clinics, referral clinics and semen testing laboratories
- The recruitment of registered survivors to help with the delivery of health and other services, for example, peer educators for the enrolment of men in screening programmes for semen testing and involvement of survivors in blood and plasma donations

- Provide counselling, advice on safe sex and condom use to prevent the spread of the virus in survivors to other people through sexual contact
- Social support through self-help groups and networking of parents and children dealing with the long-term implications microcephaly and other physical complications
- Counselling, self-help groups and networking of to address the consequences of stigma, loss of income and social isolation
- Advice to pregnant women about access to technology for detecting Zika virus infection and, if such is the case, access to counselling and psychosocial advice
- Social support for patients with severe Guillain–Barré syndrome

# Glossary

| | |
|---|---|
| Bottom-up | An approach to help people to identify and then act on their own needs. |
| Case definition | A set of diagnostic criteria that must be fulfilled to identify a particular disease and that is based on clinical, laboratory, epidemiological or combined criteria. |
| Civil-military coordination | The coordination, in support of a mission, between a military authority and civil actors, local authorities, international and non-governmental organisations. |
| Clinical trial | A research study that prospectively assigns human participants to one or more health-related interventions to evaluate the effects on health outcomes. Clinical trials are commonly classified into distinct phases. |
| Cluster | A group of organisations interconnected by their respective mandates and that work together towards common objectives. |
| Communicable (infectious or transmissible) disease | A clinically evident illness resulting from pathogenic agents in a population including viruses, bacteria and protozoa and transmitted from a source such as from a human or an animal vector to another person. |
| Communication for development (C4D) | A social process based on building a dialogue using a broad range of tools and methods towards sustained and meaningful change. |
| Conflict resolution | Facilitation of the peaceful ending of conflict between individuals or groups by actively communicating information about their different motives or ideologies and by engaging in collective negotiation. |

| | |
|---|---|
| Counselling | An interaction in which someone seeks to explore, understand or resolve a problem or a troubling personal aspect that is preventing them from living their lives in a way that they would wish to do so. |
| Crisis communication (also known as emergency communication) | Organisation, analysis, planning, decision-making and assignment of available resources to mitigate, prepare for, respond to and protect property and the environment when a health emergency occurs. |
| Disease outbreak | The occurrence of cases of disease in excess of what would normally be expected in a defined community, geographical area or season. |
| Drug resistance | The reduction in effectiveness of a drug in treating a disease because of the resistance by some pathogens. |
| Empowerment | A process by which individuals, families and communities gain more control over the decisions and resources that influence their lives and health. |
| Epidemiology | The study of the patterns, causes and effects of health and disease conditions in defined populations; identifying risk factors for disease and preventive health care goals. |
| Fear based | An intervention that uses the threat of harmful consequences to the target audience for their starting or continuing a particular high-risk behaviour. |
| Health emergency | The consequences of events on health including natural disasters, disease outbreaks and the release of hazardous materials into the environment. |
| Health promotion | A process of enabling people to increase control over, and to improve, their lives in a disease outbreak or health emergency. |
| Humanitarian crisis | A profound social crisis which is characterised by high numbers of casualties, a large scale of internal and external displacement and widespread hunger and disease. |
| Knowledge, attitude and practice (KAP) | A representation of a specific population by collecting information on or influencing what is known (knowledge), believed (attitude) and done (practice) in relation to a particular health behaviour. |

| | |
|---|---|
| Mapping | The identification, ranking and prioritisation of assets; the causes of problems and the solutions to resolve them. |
| Notifiable disease | A disease that, by statutory requirements, must be reported to the public health authorities. |
| Peer education | Promoting health-enhancing changes among and by peers rather than by health professionals educating members of the public. |
| Quarantine | An intervention, which may be enforced or self-imposed, to separate and restrict the movement of persons. |
| Rapid assessment | New information is collected quickly to meet the requirements of rapidly changing circumstances to provide reliable and quantified data. |
| Risk communication | An interactive process of exchange of information and opinion on risk usually among risk assessors, risk managers and other interested stakeholders. |
| Risk factor | A social, economic or biological status, behaviour or environment which is associated with or cause increased susceptibility to a specific disease, to ill health or an injury. |
| Rumour | An unverified but relevant statement of information spread among people and caused by gaps in knowledge, by traditional beliefs and negative experiences of health service delivery. |
| Screening | The early identification of disease to enable prevention and treatment to reduce mortality from communicable diseases. |
| Social mobilisation | The process of engaging with and motivating people to collectively achieve better health and lives. |
| Stigma | The consequences of processes that brand someone as different in ways that can result in discrimination, loss of status and social exclusion. |
| Super-spreader | A host, such as a human, that is infected with a disease and that in turn infects disproportionally more secondary contacts than other hosts also infected with the same disease. |

| | |
|---|---|
| Surveillance | The collection of information from many sources, including reported cases of diseases, hospital admissions, laboratory reports, population surveys, employment records and reported causes of death for the purpose of disease prevention and control. |
| Top-down | An approach that identifies health needs by the 'top' structures and then delivers these 'down' to others often at the community level. |
| Volunteering | An activity that involves spending time doing something for free and that aims to benefit others including relatives and friends. |
| Zoonotic | A disease that can be transmitted from animals to people or, more specifically, is a disease that normally exists in animals but that can also infect humans. |

# References

Action Against Hunger. (2013). *Conducting KAP Surveys: A Learning Document Based on KAP Failures.* http://www.actionagainsthunger.org/about/acf-international, Accessed 29/8/2016.

Adetunji, H. (2008). Principles of epidemiology in key concepts in public health. In Wilson, F., Mabhala, A., (eds.). *Key Concepts in Public Health.* Part 1. Chapter 7. London: Sage.

Albarracin, D., Gillette, J., Earl, A., Glasman, L.R., Durantini, M.R., Ho, M-H. (2005). A test of major assumptions about behaviour change: A comprehensive look at the effects of passive and active HIV-prevention interventions since the beginning of the epidemic. *Psychological Bulletin* 131(6): 856–897.

Ali, M., Lopez, A.L., You, Y.A. (2012). The global burden of cholera. *Bulletin World Health Organization* 90: 209.

Allmark, P., Tod, A. (2006). How should public health professionals engage with lay epidemiology? *Journal of Medical Ethics* 32: 460–463.

Allsop, J., Jones, K., Baggott, R. (2004). Health consumer groups in the UK: A new social movement. *Sociology of Health & Illness* 26(6): 737–756.

Almedom, A., Tumwine, J. (2008). Resilience to disasters: A paradigm shift from vulnerability to strength. *African Health Sciences* 8(Suppl 1): 1–4.

Amazigo, U. (2008). The African Programme for Onchocerciasis Control (APOC). *Annals of Tropical Medicine & Parasitology* 102(Suppl 1): 19–22.

Andreasen, A.R. (1995). *Marketing Social Change.* San Francisco, CA: Jossey Bass.

Appleton, B., Sijbesma, C. (2005). *Hygiene Promotion.* Thematic overview paper 1. Delft, The Netherlands: IRC International Water and Sanitation Centre.

Araujo, E., Maeda, A. (2013). *How to Recruit and Retain Health Workers in Rural and Remote Areas in Developing Countries.* Health, Nutrition and Population (HNP) discussion paper. Washington, DC: World Bank.

Armed Conflict Location and Event Data Project (ACLED). (2014). *Conflict Trends (No. 31): Real Time Analysis of African Political Violence.* October 2014. pp. 14–15.

Assessment Capacities Project (ACAPS). (2015). *Ebola Outbreak in West Africa Lessons Learned from Quarantine – Sierra Leone and Liberia.* 19 March 2015.

Avery-Gomez, E. (2008). Connecting communities of need with public health: can sms text-messaging improve outreach communication? *Hawaii International Conference on System Sciences, Proceedings of the 41st Annual conference.* 7–10 January 2008.

Bah, C. (2015). *The Ebola Outbreak in West Africa: Corporate Gangsters, Multinationals and Rogue Politicians.* Philadelphia, PA: Africanist Press.

Bah-Wakefield, K. (2015). *Report of the Social Anthropologist.* Ebola Response. Sierra Leone: World Health Organization country office. January/February 2015.

Bedford, J. (2014). *The Flow of Money at the Community Level: Key Considerations.* Accra, Ghana: United Nations Mission for Ebola Emergency Response. 15 November 2014.

Bell-Woodard, G., Chad, K., Labonte, R., and Martin, L., (2005). *Community capacity assessment of an active living health promotion program – Saskatoon in Motion.* Saskatoon, Saskatchewan: University of Saskatchewan.

Bertrand, J., Merritt, A., Saffitz, G. (2011). Health communication: A catalyst to behaviour change. In Parker, R., Sommer, M., (eds.). *Routledge Handbook of Global Public Health.* Chapter 31. Abingdon, UK: Routledge.

Bhattacharya, K., Winch, P., LeBan, K., Tien, M. (2001). *Community Health Workers. Incentives and Disincentives: How They Affect Motivation, Retention and Sustainability.* Published by the Basic Support for Institutionalizing Child Survival Project (BASICS II) for the United States Agency for International Development. Arlington, Virginia.

Birungi, J., Anand, S., Kinyanjui, J., Chatterjee, A., Alam, M., Mutai, C., Kemoh, S. (2016). *Use of SMS-Based Platforms for Health Communication and Monitoring in the Context of Polio Outbreak Response.* New York: UNICEF. 31 May 2016.

Brennan, B., Gutierrez, V. (2011). *Field Guide for Developing a Risk Communication Strategy.* Geneva: PAHO/WHO.

Brennan, L., Binney, W. (2010). Fear-based, guilt and shame campaigns in social marketing. *Journal of Business Research* 63(2): 14–146.

Britten, N. (1995). Qualitative interviews in medical research. *British Medical Journal* 311: 251–253.

Burgess, H., Maiese, M. (2004). Rumour control. Beyond intractability. In Burgess, G., Burgess, H., (eds.). *Conflict Information Consortium.* Boulder: University of Colorado.

Burgess, R.G. (1982). *Field Research: A Source Book and Field Manual.* London: Allen & Unwin.

Cabinet Office (UK). (2011). *Communicating Risk Guidance: Improving the UK's Ability to Absorb, Respond To and Recover From Emergencies.* London: UK Cabinet Office.

CAFOD. (2015). *Keeping the Faith: The Role of Faith Leaders in the Ebola Response.* CAFOD, Christian Aid, Islamic Relief Worldwide and Tearfund. http://cafod.org.uk/, Accessed 15/2/2017.

Cass, A., Lowell, A., Christie, M., Snelling, P.L., Flack, M., Marrnganyin, B., Brown, I. (2002). Sharing the true stories: Improving communication between aboriginal patients and health care workers. *The Medical Journal of Australia* 176(10): 466–470.

Center for Communication Programs. (2014). *Social and Behaviour Change Communication*. Baltimore, MD: Center for communication programs, Johns Hopkins University.

Center for Disaster Preparedness (CDP). (2015). *Mainstreaming Community-Based Mitigation in City Governance Community-Based Disaster Risk Management & Local Governance. Good Practices and Lessons Learned in the Philippines*. Quezon City, Philippines.

Centers of Disease Control and Prevention (CDC). (2012). *Crisis and Emergency Risk Communication*. Atlanta, GA: CDC.

Centers of Disease Control and Prevention (CDC). (2016). *Prevention Steps for a Person Who is Confirmed to Have, or Being Evaluated For, MERS-CoV Infection*. Atlanta, GA. http://www.cdc.gov/coronavirus/mers/hcp/home-care-patient.html. Accessed 12/2/2017.

Centers for Disease Control and Prevention (CDC). (2017). *Prevention and Treatment of Avian Influenza A Viruses in People*. https://www.cdc.gov/flu/avianflu/prevention.htm, Accessed 1/3/2017.

Chambers, R. (1997). *Whose Reality Counts? Putting the First Last*. London: Intermediate Technology Publications.

Chanda, E., Govere, J., Macdonald, M., Lako, R., Haque, U., Baba, S., Mnzava, A. (2013). Integrated vector management: A critical strategy for combating vector-borne diseases in South Sudan. *Malaria Journal* 12: 369.

Chandler, C., Fairhead, J., Kelly, A., Leach, M., Martineau, F., Mokuwa, E., Parker, M., Richards, P., Wilkinson, A. (2014). Ebola: Limitations of correcting misinformation. *The Lancet* 385(9975): 1275–1277. Published Online December 19, 2014. http://dx.doi.org/10.1016/S0140-6736(14)62382-5.

Christakis, N.A., Fowler, J.H. (2007). The spread of obesity in a large social network over 32 years. *New England Journal of Medicine* 357(4): 370–379.

Coghlan, B., Brennan, R., Ngov, P., Dofara, D., Ottoa, B., Clements, M., Stewart, T. (2006). Mortality in the Democratic Republic of Congo: A nationwide survey. *The Lancet* 367(9504): 44–51.

Coleman, P.T. (2000). Power and conflict. In Deutsch, M., Coleman, P.T., (eds.). *The Handbook of Conflict Resolution. Theory and Practice*. San Francisco, CA: Jossey-Bass.

Committee on Risk Perception and Communication. (1989). *Improving Risk Communication*. Washington, DC: National Academy Press.

Corcoran, N. (ed.). (2013). *Communicating Health: Strategies for Health Promotion* (2nd edition). London: Sage.

Covello, V., Allen, F. (1998). *Seven Cardinal Rules of Risk Communication*. Washington, DC: Environmental Protection Agency.

Crosier, S. (2012). *John Snow: The London Cholera Epidemic of 1854*. Center for spatially integrated socially science. http://www.csiss.org/classics, Accessed 14/5/2012.

Curtis, V., Kanki, B., Cousens, S., Diallo, I., Kpozehouen, A., Sangare, M., Nikiema, M. (2001). Evidence of behaviour change following a hygiene promotion programme in Burkina Faso. *Bulletin of the World Health Organization* 79(6): 518–527.

Cwikel, J.G. (2006). *Social Epidemiology: Strategies for Public Health Activism.* New York: Columbia University Press.

Dalling, M., Bangura, M. (2014). *Draft Concept Note: Ebola Viral Disease Survivors Conference.* UNICEF. 9 October 2014.

Dhillon, R.S., Kelly, J.D. (2015). Community Trust and the Ebola Endgame. *The New England Journal of Medicine* 373(9): 787–789.

DiFonzo, N., Bordia, P. (2007). Rumor, gossip and urban legends. *Diogenes* 54(1): 19–35.

Doctors Without Borders. (2015). *Tanzania: MSF Vaccinates 130,000 Refugees Against Cholera.* 30th July. http://www.doctorswithoutborders.org/article/tanzania-msf-vaccinates-130000-refugees-against-cholera, Accessed 25/10/2016.

Doherty, P. (2013). *Pandemics: What Everyone Needs to Know.* Oxford: Oxford University Press.

Dormandy, E., Michie, S., Weinman, J., Marteau, T. (2002). Variation in uptake of serum screening: The role of service delivery. *Prenatal Diagnosis* 22(1): 67–69.

Drexler, J.F., Corman, V.M., Gloza-Rausch, F., Seebens, A., Annan, A. (2009). Henipavirus RNA in African bats. *PLoS One* 4(7): e6367.

Dryden, W., Feltham, C. (1993). *Brief Counselling: A Practical Guide for Beginning Practitioners.* Milton Keynes: Open University Press.

Ebola Response Anthropology Platform. (2014). *Stigma and Ebola: An Anthropological Approach to Understanding and Addressing Stigma Operationally in the Ebola Response.* Policy briefing paper. 27 November 2014.

Ebola Response Anthropology Platform. (2014a). *Ebola Survivors: Using A Step Wise Re-Integration Process to Establish Social Contracts between Survivors and Their Home Communities.* Concept note. http://www.ebola-anthropology.net/05/12/2014, Accessed 12/11/2016

Enria, L., Lees, S., Smout, E., Mooney, T., Tengbeh, A., Leigh, B., Greenwood, B., Watson-Jones, D., Larson, H. (2016). Power, fairness and trust: Understanding and engaging with vaccine trial participants and communities in the setting up the EBOVAC-Salone vaccine trial in Sierra Leone. *BMC Public Health* 16: 1140. http://dx.doi.org/10.1186/s12889-016-3799-x.

Fairhead, J. (2014). *The Significance of Death, Funerals and The After-Life in Ebola-Hit Sierra Leone, Guinea and Liberia: Anthropological Insights into Infection and Social Resistance.* Brighton: Sussex University.

Falkirk council/HealthProm. (2013). *You've Got a Friend In Me. Befriending and Volunteer Scheme Handbook.* London: Healthprom.

Folayan, M.O., Yakubu, A., Haire, B., Peterson, K. (2016). Ebola vaccine development plan: Ethics, concerns and proposed measures. *BMC Medical Ethics* 17: 10. http://dx.doi.org/10.1186/s12910-016-0094-4.

Forsyth, D., R. (2009). *Group Dynamics* (5th edition). Singapore: Cengage Learning.

Freire, P. (2005). *Education for Critical Consciousness*. New York: Continuum Press.

Frusciante, A.K. (2007). Leadership, participatory democratic. In Andersen, G.L., Herr, K.G., (eds.). *Encyclopedia of Activism and Social Justice*. London: Sage.

Gallagher, J. (2017). *Ebola 'Super-Spreaders' Cause Most Cases.* 14th February 2017. http://www.bbc.co.uk/news/health-38955871, Accessed 26/2/2017.

George Washington University. (2014). *The Ebola Response. Preliminary Guidance and Recommendations.* The AAA/Wenner-Gren Ebola Emergency Response Workshop. 6–7th November 2014.

Gillespie, A.M., Obregon, R., Asawi, R.E., Richey, C., Manoncourt, E., Joshi, K., Naqvi, S., et al. (2016). Social mobilization and community engagement central to the Ebola response in West Africa: Lessons for future public health emergencies. *Global Health, Science and Practice* 4(4): 626–646. http://dx.doi.org/10.9745/GHSP-D-16-00226.

Gilmore, G. (2011). *Needs and Capacity Assessment for Health Education and Health Promotion* (4th edition). Boston, MA: Jones and Bartlett Learning.

Ginsberg, P. E. (1988). Evaluation in cross-cultural perspective. *Evaluation and Program Planning* 11: 189–195.

Glesne, C., Peshkin, A. (1992). *Becoming Qualitative Researchers*. New York: Longman Publishing Group.

Global Polio Eradication Initiative. (2016). *Strategy.* http://www.polioeradication.org/Aboutus/Strategy.aspx, Accessed 29/9/2016.

Goodman, R., Speers, M., McLeroy, K., Fawcett, S., Kegler, M., Parker, E., Smith, S.R., Sterling, T.D., Wallerstein, N. (1998). Identifying and defining the dimensions of community capacity to provide a base for measurement. *Health Education and Behaviour* 25(3): 258–278.

Greyling, C., Maulit, J.A., Parry, S., Robinson, D., Smith, S., Street, A., Vitillo, R. (2016). Lessons from the faith-driven response to the West Africa Ebola epidemic. *The Review of Faith & International Affairs* 14(3): 118–123. http://dx.doi.org/10.1080/15570274.2016.1215829.

Grier, S., and Bryant, C. (2005). Social marketing in public health. *Annual review of Public Health* 26: 319–339.

Guba, E.G., Lincoln, Y.S. (1989). *Fourth Generation Evaluation*. Newbury Park, CA: Sage.

Gubrium, A. (2009). Digital storytelling: An emergent method for health promotion research and practice. *Health Promotion Practice* 10(2): 186–191.

Healthcompass. (2017). *How to Conduct Qualitative Formative Research.* http://www.thehealthcompass.org/how-to-guides/how-conduct-qualitative-formative-research, Accessed 7/1/2017.

Health Protection Network. (2008). *Communicating with the Public about Health Risks. Health Protection Network Guidance 1.* Health Protection Scotland, Glasgow.

Hewlett, B.S., Hewlett, B.L. (2008). *Ebola, Culture, and Politics: The Anthropology of An Emerging Disease.* Belmont, CA: Thomson Higher Education.

Heymann, D. (2015). Ebola: Burying the bodies. *The Lancet* 385: 2455–2456.

Hinyard, L., Kreuter, M. (2006). Using narrative communication as a tool for health behavior change: A conceptual, theoretical, and empirical overview. *Health Education & Behavior* 34(5): 777–792.

Hoffman, T., Bennett, S., Del Mar, C. (2013). *Evidence–Based Practice Across the Health Professions* (2nd edition). Edinburgh: Churchill Livingstone.

Hunt, K., Emslie, C. (2001). Commentary: The prevention paradox in lay epidemiology – Rose revisited. *International Journal of Epidemiology* 30(3): 442–446.

Institute of Development Studies (IDS). (2015). *Local Engagement in Ebola Outbreaks and Beyond in Sierra Leone.* Practice paper in brief 24. February 2015.

International Centre for Aids Care and Treatment Programs (ICAP). (2015). *Rapid Mixed Methods Assessment of the Ebola Community Care Center Model in Sierra Leone.* New York: Columbia University.

International Organization for Migration (IOM). (2015). *Management of Cross-Border Movements of Frontier Communities in Mauritania.* Geneva: International Organization for Migration. http://www.iom.int/about-iom, Accessed 12/2/2017.

International Red Cross (IRC). (2013). *PHAST Approach.* International Water and Sanitation Centre. http://www.irc.nl/, Accessed 12/2/2017.

Internews. (2015). *Supporting Local Voices in the Ebola Response.* Monrovia, Liberia: Internews. 21st April 2015.

Jiang, H., Shi, G., Tu, W., Zheng, C., Lai, X., Li, X., Wi, Q., et al. (2016). Rapid assessment of knowledge, attitudes, practices, and risk perception related to the prevention and control of Ebola virus disease in three communities of Sierra Leone. *Infectious Diseases of Poverty* 5: 53.

Jirojwong, S., Liamputtong, P. (eds.). (2009). *Population Health, Communities and Health Promotion.* London: Oxford University Press.

Johnson, N. (2006). *Britain and the 1918–19 Influenza Pandemic: A Dark Epilogue.* London and New York: Routledge.

Kamradt-Scott, A., Harman, S., Wenham, C., Smith, F. (2015). *Saving Lives: The Civil-Military Response to the 2014 Ebola Outbreak in West Africa.* Sydney, Australia: University of Sydney.

Kant, I., Gregor, M., Reath, A. (1997). *Kant: Critique of Practical Reason.* Cambridge: Cambridge University Press.

Kelly, J.A., St Lawrence, J.S., Stevenson, L.Y., Hauth, A.C., Kalichman, S.C., Diaz, Y.E., Brasfield, T.L., Koob, J.J., Morgan, M.G. (1992). Community AIDS/HIV risk reduction: The effects of endorsements by popular people in three cities. *American Journal of Public Health* 82(11): 1483–1489.

Kelsey, J.L., Thompson, W.D., Evans, A.S. (1986). *Methods in Observational Epidemiology.* New York: Oxford University Press.

Kitzinger, J. (1995). Introducing focus groups. *British Medical Journal* 311: 299–302.

Kotler, P. (2000). *Marketing Management.* Upper Saddle River, NJ: Prentice Hall.

Labonte, R., Laverack, G. (2001). Capacity building in health promotion, Part 1: For whom? And for what purpose? *Critical Public Health* 11(2): 111–128.

Labonte, R., Laverack, G. (2008). *Health Promotion in Action: From Local to Global Empowerment.* London: Palgrave Macmillan.

Lamond, E., Kinjanyui, J. (2012). *Cholera Outbreak Guidelines. Preparedness, Prevention and Control.* Oxford: Oxfam.

Laverack, G. (1999). *Addressing the contradiction between discourse and practice in health promotion,* unpublished PhD thesis, Deakin University, Melbourne.

Laverack, G. (2004). *Health Promotion Practice: Power and Empowerment.* London: Sage.

Laverack, G. (2007). *Health Promotion Practice: Building Empowered Communities.* London: Open University Press.

Laverack, G. (2009). *Public Health: Power, Empowerment & Professional Practice* (2nd edition). London: Palgrave Macmillan.

Laverack, G. (2013). *A to Z of Health Promotion.* London: Palgrave.

Laverack, G. (2013a). *Health Activism: Foundations and Strategies.* London: Sage.

Laverack, G. (2014). *A to Z of Health Promotion.* Basingstoke: Palgrave Macmillan.

Laverack, G. (2015). *Public Health: Power, Empowerment & Professional Practice* (3rd edition). London: Palgrave Macmillan.

Laverack, G., Brown, K.M. (2003). Qualitative research in a cross-cultural context: Fijian experiences. *Qualitative Health Research* 13(3): 1–10.

Laverack, G., Manoncourt, E. (2015). Key experiences of community engagement and social mobilization in the Ebola response. *Global Health Promotion* 23(1): 79–82.

Leach, F. (1994). Expatriates as agents of cross-cultural transmission. *Compare: A Journal of Comparative and International Education* 24(3): 217–231.

Lennon, R., Rentfro, R., O'Leary, B. (2010). Social marketing and distraction during behaviors among young adults: The effectiveness of fear-based campaigns. *Academy of Marketing Studies Journal* 14(2): 95–113.

Lewis, S. (2016). Emergency planning and response: Working in partnership. In Sellwood, C., Wapling, A., (eds.). *Health Emergency Preparedness and Response.* Chapter 5. Wallingford: CAB International publications.

Lo Presti, A., Cella, E., Giovanetti,M., Lai, A., Angeletti, S., Zehender, G., Ciccozzi, M. (2015). Origin and evolution of Nipah virus. *Journal of Medical Virology* 88(3): 380–388. http://dx.doi.org/10.1002/jmv.24345.

Luby, S., Gurley, E., Hossain, J. (2009). Transmission of human infection with Nipah virus. *Clinical Infectious Diseases* 49(11): 1743–1748.

Luthi, E. (2015). *Quick Action to Contain Cholera.* http://www.unicef.org/infobycountry/burundi_82458.html, Accessed 29/9/2016.

Maes, B. (2014). *Polio Eradication and Immunisation: Mobilising and Engaging Communities through Radio Game Shows.* UNICEF. http://www.comminit.com/polio/content/polio-eradication-and-immunisation-mobilising-and-engaging-communities-through-radio-gam, Accessed 17/9/2016.

Maibach, E.W., Rothschild, M.L., Novelli, W.D. (2002). Social marketing. In Glanz, K., Rimer, B.K., Lewis, F.M., (eds.). *Health Behavior and Health Education: Theory, Research, and Practice* (3rd edition). San Franciso, CA: Jossey Bass. pp. 347–361.

Marks, D. (2002). *Perspectives on Evidence-Based Practice*. London: Health Development Agency. Public health evidence steering group. Project 00477.

Marshall, K., Smith, S. (2015). Religion and Ebola: Learning from experience. *The Lancet* 386: E24–E25.

Martin, B. (2007). Activism, social and political. In Andersen, G.L., Herr, K.G., (eds.). *Encyclopedia of Activism and Social Justice*. London: Sage.

Mays, N., Pope, C. (1995). Observational methods in health care settings. *British Medical Journal* 311: 182–184.

McConnell, T. (2014). *Some people would rather die of Ebola than stop hugging sick loved ones*. Global Post, 10 October 2014. http://www.globalpost.com/dispatch/news/health/141010/familes-cant-mourn-ebola-victims-liberia, Accessed 25/8/2016.

McCreadie, R., Macdonald, C., Ounis, L. (2015). *Crowdsourced Rumour Identification during Emergencies*. University of Glasgow, UK. International World Wide Web Conference Committee.

McLeod, J., and Mcleod, J. (2011). *A Practical Guide for Counsellors and Helping Professionals*. London, UK: Open University Press.

Medecins Sans Frontieres (MSF). (2015). *Pushed to the Limit and Beyond A Year into the Largest Ever Ebola Outbreak*. Geneva, Switzerland. http://www.msf.org, Accessed 25/11/2016.

Minichiello, V., Aroni, R., Timewell, E., Alexander, L. (1990). *Indepth Interviewing. Researching People*. Southbank, Victoria, Australia: Longman Cheshire.

Ministry of Health. (2015). *Getting to Zero National Campaign 2015. Let's End This Together – Leh we Tap Ebola*. Freetown, Sierra Leone: Ministry of Health.

Mitchell, C., Banks, M. (1998). *Handbook of Conflict Resolution. The Analytical Problem-Solving Approach*. London: Pinter.

Muzundar, T. (2017). *Vaccines for Three Deadly Viruses Fast-Tracked*. 18th January. BBC World News. http://www.bbc.co.uk/news/health-38669584, Accessed 17/3/2017.

Naidoo, J., Wills, J. (2009). *Foundations for Health Promotion* (3rd edition). Edinburgh: Bailliere and Tindall.

National Health Service (NHS). (2017). *Bird Flu (Avian Flu) – Prevention*. http://www.nhs.uk/Conditions/Avian-flu/Pages/Prevention.aspx, Accessed 1/3/2017.

National Research Council. (2003). *The Resistance Phenomenon in Microbes and Infectious Disease Vectors: Implications for Human Health and Strategies for Containment*. Washington, DC: The National Academies Press.

Needham, C., Hoang, T.K., Nguyen, V.H., Le, D.C., Michael, E., Drake, L., Hall, A., Bundy, A.P. (1998). Epidemiology of soil-transmitted nematode infections in Ha Nam Province, Vietnam. *Tropical Medicine and International Health* 3(11): 904–912.

Nelson, D., Adger, R., Brown, K. (2007). Adaptation to environmental change: Contributions of a resilience framework. *The Annual Review of Environment and Resources* 32: 395–419.

Network of Public Health Observatories. (2013). Health Profiles. http://www.apho.org.uk/, Accessed 22/1/2016.

Nutbeam, D., Bauman, A. (2011). *Evaluation In a Nutshell. A Practical Guide to the Evaluation of Health Promotion Programs*. 3rd edition. London: McGraw-Hill.

Office for the Coordination of Humanitarian Affairs (OCHA). (2015). Strengthening border surveillance between Ebola affected countries. *Ebola Bulletin*. July 2015.

Oneindia. (2010). *Indian American Activists Protest*. http://news.oneindia.in, Accessed 15/6/2010.

Partners' Meeting Monrovia. (2014). *Response to Ebola Virus Disease (EVD) in Lofa County, Experiences from the Field*. Monrovia. 11th October 2014.

Pescosolido, B.A. (1991). Illness careers and network ties: A conceptual model of utilization and compliance. In Albrecht, G., Levy, J., (eds.). *Advances in Medical Sociology*. Greenwich, CT: JAI Press. pp. 161–184.

PLAN. (2016). *Control measures of Aedes aegypti: Focus groups research in Recife and Campina Grande*. Avaliacado monitoramento pesquisa social. Sao Paulo, Brazil.

Plows, A. (2007). Strategies and tactics in social movements. In Andersen, G.L., Herr, K.G., (eds.). *Encyclopedia of Activism and Social Justice*. London: Sage.

Porta, M. (ed) (2014). *A dictionary of epidemiology* (6th edition). Oxford, UK: Oxford University Press.

PREVENT. (2011). *Risk Communication Planning and Action Guide*. Washington, DC: USAID.

Prue, C. (2016). *Puerto Rican Pregnant Women's Assessment of Vector Control Strategies and Personal Protective Behaviors for Zika prevention*. Preliminary Report. International Risk Communication Partners Group. 11th April 2016.

Public Health Agency of Canada (PHAC). (2013). *Glossary of Terms*. http://www.phac-aspc.gc.ca/php-psp/ccph-cesp/glos-eng.php#h, Accessed 21/1/2013.

Public Health England (PHE). (2016). *Risk assessment of Middle East Respiratory Syndrome Coronavirus (MERS-CoV)*. PHE, London. Update March 2016. https://www.gov.uk/government/collections/middle-east-respiratory-syndrome-coronavirusmers-cov-clinical-management-and-guidance, Accessed 20/10/2016.

Raffle, A.E., Muir Gray, J.A. (2007). *Screening – Evidence and Practice*. Oxford: Oxford University Press.

Rashid, I. (2012). *Epidemic and Resistance in Sierra Leone*. http://www.academia.edu/2350892/Epidemic_and_Resistance_in_Sierra_Leone, Accessed 27/8/2016.

Reuters. (2014). *Ebola Center in Sierra Leone under Guard after Protest March*. 27th July 2014. http://af.reuters.com/article/topNews/idAFKBN0FW04D20140727.

Reynolds, B., Crouse-Quinn, S. (2008). Effective communication during an influenza pandemic: The value of using a crisis and emergency risk communication framework. *Health Promotion Practice* 9(4 suppl): 13S–17S.

Richards, P. (2015). Village responses to Ebola virus disease. In *Rural Sierra Leone. An Analytical Overview*. Sierra Leone: Social Mobilisation Action Consortium.

Roberts, L. (2015). As Ebola fades, a new threat. *Science* 347(6227): 1189. http://dx.doi.org/10.1126/science.347.6227.1189.

Rosato, M., Laverack, G., Howard Grabman, L., Tripathy, P., Nair, N., Mwansambo, C., Azad, K., et al. (2008). Alma Ata: Rebirth and revision 5: Community participation: Lessons for maternal, newborn and child health. *The Lancet* 372(9642): 962–972.

Rothman, K., Greenland, S., Lash, T. (2008). *Modern Epidemiology* (3rd edition). Philadelphia, PA: Lippincott, Williams & Wilkins. p. 561.

Russon, C. (1995). The influence of culture on evaluation. *Evaluation Journal of Australasia* 7(1): 44–49.

Rychetnik, L., Wise, M. (2004). Advocating evidence-based health promotion: Reflections and a way forward. *Health Promotion International* 19(2): 247–257.

Sahr Sahidn, J. (2015). *Pros and cons of Sierra Leone's Ebola lockdowns. Integrated Regional Information Networks*. 9th April 2015.

Sechrest, L.E. (1997). Book review. Empowerment evaluation: Knowledge and tools for self-assessment & accountability. *Environment and Behavior* 29(3): 422–426.

Seefeldt, F.M. (1985). Cultural considerations for evaluation consulting in the Egyptian context. In Patton, M.Q., (ed.). *Culture and Evaluation*. San Francisco, CA: Jossey-Bass. pp. 69–78.

Sierra Leone Emergency Management Program. (2014). *Standard Operating Procedure for Community Engagement with Reference to the Ebola Community Care Units*. Freetown, Sierra Leone: Ministry of Health.

Seiter, R.H., Gass, J.S. (2010). *Persuasion, Social Influence, and Compliance Gaining* (4th edition). Boston, MA: Allyn & Bacon.

Shen, Z., Ning, F., Zhou, W., He, X., Lin, C., Chin, D.P., Zhu, Z., Schuchat, A. (2004). Super-spreading SARS events: Beijing 2003. *Emerging Infectious Diseases* 10(2): 256–260.

Smith, R. (2002). The discomfort of patient power. *British Medical Journal* 324: 497–498.

Smithies, J., Webster, G. (1998). *Community Involvement in Health*. Aldershot, England: Ashgate Publishing Ltd.

Social Mobilisation Action Consortium (SMAC). (2014). *Community-Led Ebola Action (CLEA): Field Guide for Community Mobilizers*. Freetown, Sierra Leone.

South, J., White, J., Gamsu, M. (2013). *People-Centred Public Health*. University of Bristol, Bristol: Policy Press.

Srinivasan, L. (1993). *Tools for Community Participation. A Manual for Training Trainers in Participatory Techniques*. New York: PROWWESS/UNDP.

Stewart, A. (2013). *Lets-get-ready-planning-together-emergencies*. http://comminit.com/global/content/, Accessed 29/9/2016.

Stewart, M.A., Brown, J.B., Weston, W.W., McWhinney, I.R., McWilliam, C.L., Freeman, T.R. (2003). *Patient Centred Medicine: Transforming the Clinical Method* (2nd edition). Oxford: Radcliffe Medical Publications.

Taylor, R., Rieger, A. (1985). Medicine as a social science: Rudolf Virchow on the typhus epidemic in Upper Silesia. *International Journal of Health Services* 15: 547–559.

Tellier, S., Roche, N. (2016). *Public Health in Humanitarian Action.* Copenhagen: School of Global Health, University of Copenhagen.

Tengland, P. (2013). Behavior change or empowerment: On the ethics of health promotion goals. *Health Care Analysis* 24(1): 24–46. Published online 8/10/2013.

The Guardian. (2016). *Yellow Fever in Congo: MSF Vaccinates 710,000 People in Ten Days.* 12th September 2016. https://www.theguardian.com/global-development/gallery/2016/sep/12/yellow-fever-democratic-republic-congo-msf-vaccinates-710000-people-10-days-kinshasa-in-pictures, Accessed 15/3/2017.

Thomas, P. (2001). Empowering community health: Women in Samoa. In Pencheorn, D., Guest, C., Melzer, D., Muir Gray J.A., (eds.). *Oxford Handbook of Public Health Practice.* Oxford: Oxford University Press.

Thomas, S., Olds, T., Pettigrew, S., Yeatman, H., Hyde, J., Dragovic, C. (2014). Parent and child reactions with two contrasting anti-obesity advertising campaigns: A qualitative analysis. *BMC Public Health* 14(151): 1–11.

Trinh, H.V., Luong, X.H., Hoang, T.L., Le, T.T., Nuygen, D.H., Le, D.C., Ta, H.T., Doan, T.T., Nuygen, N.T. (1999). *KAP Study on School Sanitation and Control of Worm Infection.* Ministry of Health. Thai Binh Medical College, Thai Binh, Vietnam.

UNAIDS. (2007). *Good Participatory Practice Guidelines for Biomedical HIV Prevention Trials.* UNAIDS/07.30E/JC1364E. Geneva: UNAIDS.

UNDP. (2002). *Communication Behaviour Change Tools.* Entertainment-Education. volume 1. pp. 1–6. New York: UNDP.

UNICEF. (1999). *A Manual on Health Promotion.* Water, Environment and sanitation technical guidelines. Series 6. New York.

UNICEF. (2013). *Peer Education.* http://www.unicef.org/lifeskills/index_12078.html, Accessed 21/10/2016.

UNICEF. (2014). *Survivor Networks in Sierra Leone.* http://www.unicef.org/cbsc/index_65736.html, Accessed 29/9/2016.

UNICEF. (2015). *Reaching Out to Root Out Ebola.* http://www.unicef.org/infobycountry/guinea_81976.html, Accessed 29/9/2016.

UNICEF. (2015a). *Social Mobilizers Empower 'Hotspot' Communities to Fight Ebola in Sierra Leone.* http://www.unicef.org/infobycountry/sierraleone_78953.html, Accessed 29/9/2016.

UNICEF. (2015b). *Tackling Cholera in Haiti.* https://blogs.unicef.org/blog/tackling-cholera-in-haiti/, Accessed 29/9/2016.

UNICEF. (2015c). *Knowledge, Attitude and Practice Survey in Ebola Survivors.* http://www.unicef.org/cbsc/index_65736.html, Accessed 29/9/2016.

UNICEF. (2016d). *Community Radio and Ebola in Guinea.* http://www.unicef.org/emergencies/ebola/75941_82520.html, Accessed 29/9/2016.

UNICEF. (2016e). *My Future is My Choice – Life Skills Programme through Peer Education in Namibia*. http://www.unicef.org/lifeskills/index_8798.html, Accessed 16/10/2016.

Volunteering England. (2012). *What is Volunteering?* http://www.volunteering.org.uk, Accessed 5/1/2014.

Waldman, R., Kruk, M. (2011). Conflict, health, and health systems: A global perspective. In Parker, R., Sommer, M., (eds.). *Routledge Handbook of Global Public Health*. Chapter 22. Abingdon, UK: Routledge.

Walker, P. and Marie, J. (2011). *From public health to wellbeing: the new driver for policy and action*. Basingstoke, UK: Palgrave Macmillan.

Walker, P., White, M., Griffin, J., Reynolds, A., Ferguson, N., Ghani, A. (2015). Malaria morbidity and mortality in Ebola-affected countries caused by decreased health-care capacity, and the potential effect of mitigation strategies: A modelling analysis. *The Lancet* 15(7): 825–832. Published online April 24, 2015. http://dx.doi.org/10.1016/S1473-3099(15)70124-6.

Warraich, H. (2009). Religious opposition to polio vaccination. *Emerging Infectious Diseases* 15(6): 978. http://dx.doi.org/10.3201/eid1506.090087.

Watts, D. (2003). *Six Degrees: The Science of a Connected Age*. London: William Heinemann publishers.

Werner, D. (1988). Empowerment and health. *Contact, Christian Medical Commission*, 102: 1–9.

White, H.C. (1992). *Identity and Control: A Structured Theory of Social Action*. Princeton, NJ: Princeton University Press.

Wigmore, R. (2016). *Contextualising Ebola rumours from a political, historical and social perspective to understand people's perceptions of Ebola and the responses to it*. University of Sussex. Ebola Response Anthropology Platform. Policy briefing paper. http://www.ebola-anthropology.net/wp-content/uploads/2015/10/Contextualising-Ebola-rumours-from-a-political.pdf, Accessed 14/11/2016.

Wilkinson, A., Leach, M. (2014). Ebola-Myths, realities and structural violence. *African Affairs* 114/454: 136–148. http://dx.doi.org/10.1093/afraf/adu08.

Winfield, M. (2013). *The Essential Volunteer Handbook*. Victoria, BC, Canada: Friesen press.

Wong, G., Liu, W., Liu, Y., Zhou, B., Bi, Y., Gao, G. (2015). MERS, SARS, and Ebola: The role of super-spreaders in infectious disease. *Cell Host and Microbe* 18(4): 398–401.

Wood, S., Sawyer, R., Simpson-Hebert, M. (1998). *PHAST Step-by-step-Guide*. Geneva: World Health Organization.

Wolff, B. (2015). *Hand-off Report: CDC Sierra Leone Ebola Response*. Atlanta, GA: Public Health Service, Centers for Disease Control.

World Congress on Communication for Development. (2007). *Lessons, Challenges and the Way Forward*. Food and Agriculture Organization of the UN and the World Bank, Rome.

World Council of Churches. (2015). *Responding to Ebola. A Health and Humanitarian Crisis*. Geneva, Switzerland: World Council of Churches.

World Health Organization. (1986). *Ottawa Charter for Health Promotion*. Geneva: World Health Organization.

World Health Organization. (1998). *The Health Promotion Glossary*. Geneva: World Health Organization.

World Health Organization. (2006). *Making Preparation Count: Lessons from the Avian Influenza Outbreak in Turkey*. Copenhagen: EURO office, World Health Organization.

World Health Organization. (2006a). *Evaluation of the Integrated Pest and Vector Management (IPVM) Project in Sri Lanka*. New Delhi: WHO Regional Office for South-East Asia. http://www.searo.who.int/en/Section23/Section1001/Section1110_12796.htm, Accessed 18/3/2017.

World Health Organization. (2006b). *The World Health Report – Working Together for Health*. Geneva: World Health Organization.

World Health Organization. (2007). *Health of indigenous Peoples. Fact sheet number 326*. Geneva: World Health Organization.

World Health Organization. (2009). *Polio Eradication Evaluation: Major Barriers to Interrupting Poliovirus Transmission*. Geneva: World Health Organization.

World Health Organization. (2009a). *Global Health Risks: Mortality and Burden of Disease Attributable to Selected Major Risks*. Geneva: World Health Organization.

World Health Organization. (2010). *The World Health Report: Health Systems Financing-the Path to Universal Coverage*. Geneva: World Health Organization.

World Health Organization. (2012). *Handbook for Integrated Vector Management*. WHO/HTM/NTD/VEM/2012.3. Geneva: World Health Organization.

World Health Organization. (2012a). *International Standards for Clinical Trial Registries*. Geneva: World Health Organization.

World Health Organization. (2014). *Interim Guidance for National Health Authorities and Blood Transfusion Services. Version 1*. Geneva: World Health Organization.

World Health Organization. (2014a). *Ebola Response Roadmap Situation Report Update*. Geneva: World Health Organization. http://www.who.int/csr/disease/ebola/situation-reports/en/?m=20141121, Accessed 26/11/2014.

World Health Organization. (2015). *How to Conduct Safe and Dignified Burial of a Patient Who has Died from Suspected or Confirmed Ebola Virus Disease*. WHO/EVD/GUIDANCE/Burials/14.2. Geneva: World Health Organization.

World Health Organization. (2015a). *Cholera. Fact sheet number 107*. Updated July 2015. Geneva: World Health Organization.

World Health Organization. (2015b). *Risk Communication*. http://www.who.int/risk-communication/photos/reaching-engaging-community/en/, Accessed 18/3/2017.

World Health Organization. (2015c). *Ebola Situation Reports*. Geneva: World Health Organization. http://www.who.int/ebola/situationreports, Accessed 9/8/2016.

World Health Organization. (2015d). *Communication and Social Mobilization in Yellow Fever Mass Vaccination Campaigns: 10 Points from Field Experience*. Geneva: World Health Organization.

World Health Organization. (2015e). *Factors that Contributed to Undetected Spread of the Ebola Virus and Impeded Rapid Containment*. http://www.who.int/csr/disease/ebola/one-year-report/factors/en/, Accessed 12/8/2016.

World Health Organization. (2015f). *Middle East Respiratory Syndrome Coronavirus (MERS-CoV)*. Fact sheet No. 401. Geneva: World Health Organization.

World Health Organization. (2016). *Ebola Situation Reports*. Geneva: World Health Organization. http://www. who.int/ebola/situationreports, Accessed 9/8/2016.

World Health Organization. (2016a). *Zika Strategic Response Plan*. Updated 30 June 2016. WHO/ZIKV/SRF/16.3. Geneva: World Health Organization.

World Health Organization. (2016b). *Chikungunya Fact sheet*. May 2016. Geneva: World Health Organization.

World Health Organization. (2016c). *Case Definitions for the Four Diseases Requiring Notification in All Circumstances Under the International Health Regulations*. Geneva: World Health Organization. http://www.who.int/ihr/Case_Definitions.pdf, Accessed 2/12/2016.

World Health Organization. (2016d). Fact sheet. *Vector-borne diseases*. Geneva: World Health Organization. http://www.who.int/mediacentre/fact-sheets/fs387/en/, Accessed 15/11/2016.

World Health Organization. (2016e). *Yellow Fever*. Fact sheet. May 2016. Geneva: World Health Organization.

World Health Organization. (2016f). *International Health Regulations 2005* (3rd edition). Geneva: World Health Organization.

World Health Organization. (2016g). *The World Health Organization Heightens the Health Response to A Cholera Outbreak*. Geneva: World Health Organization. http://www.afro.who.int/fr/republique-centrafricaine/press-materials/item/8889-who-heightens-health-response-to-cholera-outbreak-in-car.html, Accessed 11/8/2016.

World Health Organization. (2017). *Avian Influenza-China. Disease outbreak news*. http://www.who.int/csr/don/22-february-2017-ah7n9-china/en/, Accessed 22/2/2017.

World Health Organization. (2017a). *Avian and Other Zoonotic Influenza*. Fact sheet. Updated November 2016. http://www.who.int/mediacentre/fact-sheets/avian_influenza/en/, Accessed 28/2/2017.

Wright, J. (2001). Assessing health needs. In Pencheon, D., Muir Gray, J. A., Guest, C. and Melzer, D (eds). *Oxford Handbook of Public Health Practice*. Oxford, UK: Oxford University Press, pp. 38–47.

Zakus, J.D.L., Lysack, C.L. (1998). Revisiting community participation. *Health Policy and Planning* 13(1): 1–12.

# Index